THE CONFIDENT MAMA-TO-BE

Navigating Pregnancy with Ease

By

JOYCE EVEN

Table of Contents

Introduction

Welcome to "The Confident Mama-To-Be: Navigating Pregnancy with Ease," a comprehensive and empowering guide designed to support you through every step of your pregnancy journey. This book is your trusted companion, offering practical advice, emotional guidance, and a wealth of information to help you navigate the transformative experience of pregnancy with confidence, ease, and joy.

Pregnancy is a miraculous and life-altering journey, filled with a myriad of physical and emotional changes. From the moment you receive the joyful news of your impending motherhood to the awe-inspiring day when you finally hold your precious baby in your arms, this book aims to provide you with the knowledge, tools, and inspiration you need to embrace each stage of pregnancy with grace and self-assurance.

In the chapters ahead, we will delve into a wide range of topics, starting with the profound realization of the miracle growing within you. We will explore the physical and emotional transformations that occur during pregnancy, offering guidance on how to embrace these changes and foster a positive mindset throughout your journey.

Building a strong support network is crucial during this time, and we will provide you with insights into effective communication with your partner, loved ones, and healthcare professionals. Additionally, we will explore the value of connecting with other expectant mothers, creating a community of support, and sharing the joys and challenges that arise along the way.

Nurturing your body and well-being is paramount during pregnancy, and we will guide you in maintaining a healthy lifestyle through proper nutrition, exercise, and self-care practices. We will address common discomforts and provide strategies to alleviate them, ensuring your physical well-being and enhancing your overall pregnancy experience.

Emotional well-being is equally important, as hormonal changes and heightened emotions are integral aspects of the pregnancy journey. We will offer coping mechanisms for mood swings, anxiety, and fears that may arise, encouraging you to embrace mindfulness techniques, relaxation exercises, and self-reflection to foster emotional balance and harmony.

Creating a safe and nurturing environment for both yourself and your baby is a top priority, and we will guide you in preparing your home, designing a peaceful nursery, and adopting practices that promote a healthy and toxin-free environment.

Throughout the book, we emphasize the importance of bonding with your baby, exploring various ways to connect and nurture that precious relationship during pregnancy. We delve into the power of communication, touch, music, and visualization to strengthen the bond between you and your growing little one.

As you progress further into your pregnancy, we will address the practical aspects of preparing for labor and delivery. From understanding different birthing options to creating a birth plan aligned with your desires, we will provide you with the tools to make informed decisions and advocate for your preferences.

But the journey doesn't end with the arrival of your baby; it continues into the postpartum period. We will guide you in preparing for the physical and emotional changes that occur after birth, emphasizing the importance of self-care, recovery, and building a support system to navigate the challenges and joys of early motherhood.

Ultimately, this book is a celebration of your journey, highlighting the incredible strength and resilience that lies within you. It's a reminder that you are capable, powerful, and deserving of every bit of joy and fulfillment that motherhood brings. By embracing the wisdom, insights, and practical guidance found within these pages, you will embark on this beautiful adventure with confidence, grace, and a heart full of love.

So, mama-to-be, let us embark on this transformative journey together, as we navigate pregnancy with ease, embrace the joys and challenges, and celebrate the extraordinary path that leads to the precious gift of motherhood. You are not alone—this book is here to support and empower you every step of the way. Welcome to the incredible adventure of confident pregnancy!

Chapter 1: Embracing the Miracle

Discovering that you're pregnant is a truly remarkable moment in your life. It may begin with a subtle suspicion, a missed period, or a gut feeling that something has changed within you. As you hold that pregnancy test in your hands, waiting for the result, a mix of emotions floods over you—excitement, anticipation, and perhaps a touch of disbelief. And when that little plus sign or the words "pregnant" appear, a wave of joy washes over you, validating what your heart already knew: you're going to be a mother.

Embracing the Unknown

Alongside the joy, it's completely normal to experience a range of other emotions. You may feel a sense of surprise, especially if you weren't actively trying to conceive. It's okay to have worries and concerns, too. Thoughts about how your life will change, how you'll handle the responsibility of being a parent, or how your relationships may evolve are all part of the process. Remember, you're not alone in these feelings—countless mothers before you have experienced the same mix of emotions when they discovered their own pregnancies.

Connecting with Your Baby

From the moment you receive that positive result, a unique connection begins to form between you and your growing baby. While you may not be able to see or touch your little one just yet, the knowledge of their existence fills you with awe. You start to envision their tiny features, wonder about their personality, and dream about the life you'll share together. This connection deepens as you feel the first fluttering movements within your womb, a tangible reminder of the miracle taking place inside you.

As you embrace the unknown and navigate the emotions that come with discovering your pregnancy, it's important to remember that every journey is different. Your path to motherhood is uniquely yours, and there is no right or wrong way to feel. Allow yourself to experience and process these emotions at your own pace, and be gentle with yourself as you adjust to this transformative new chapter in your life.

Understanding the Physical and Emotional Changes

Hormonal Transformations

One of the first things you'll notice during pregnancy is the incredible surge of hormones coursing through your body.

Hormones such as estrogen and progesterone play vital roles in supporting the growth and development of your baby. However, these hormonal fluctuations can also lead to various physical and emotional changes.

For instance, you might experience breast tenderness and sensitivity as your body prepares for breastfeeding. Morning sickness, characterized by nausea and sometimes vomiting, is another common symptom caused by hormonal shifts. Fatigue is also prevalent in early pregnancy due to increased progesterone levels. These hormonal changes can leave you feeling exhausted and may affect your daily routine.

Navigating body changes

As your pregnancy progresses, your body will undergo remarkable transformations to accommodate the growing life within you.

Your belly will gradually expand as your baby grows, and you'll notice changes in your breasts, hips, and other areas of your body. Embracing and celebrating these changes can help you feel more connected to the process of motherhood.

Weight gain is a natural and necessary part of pregnancy as your body stores additional fat to support your baby's growth. It's essential to remember that weight gain is a positive and healthy sign. Your healthcare provider will guide you on the recommended weight gain based on your pre-pregnancy body mass index (BMI) to ensure a healthy pregnancy for both you and your baby.

A journey through trimesters

Pregnancy is divided into three trimesters, each with its own unique characteristics and milestones. The first trimester is a time of rapid development for your baby, as major organs and body systems form. During this period, you may experience symptoms like morning sickness, fatigue, and mood swings as your body adjusts to the hormonal changes.

Moving into the second trimester, you'll likely notice some relief from early pregnancy symptoms. This trimester is often referred to as the "honeymoon phase" as many women experience increased energy levels and a decrease in morning sickness. Your baby's movements, known as quickening, may also become noticeable during this time, fostering a deeper connection with your growing little one.

The third trimester brings with it a range of physical changes as your baby continues to grow and prepare for birth. Your belly will expand significantly, and you may experience increased discomfort due to the pressure on your organs and joints. Braxton Hicks contractions, which are practice contractions, may become more frequent as your body prepares for labor.

Throughout each trimester, it's important to listen to your body and communicate any concerns or discomfort with your healthcare provider. Regular prenatal check-ups will allow your healthcare team to monitor your progress, provide guidance, and address any questions or issues that arise.

Embracing the Emotional Journey

Pregnancy is not only a physical journey but an emotional one as well. Hormonal changes can contribute to heightened emotions, mood swings, and even occasional bouts of anxiety or depression. It's essential to understand that these emotional fluctuations are normal and part of the journey.

You may experience a range of emotions, from elation and excitement to moments of uncertainty or worry. Thoughts about your ability to be a good parent or concerns about the future are natural. Remember, it's okay to have these feelings, and you are not alone. Sharing your emotions with your partner, loved ones, or a support group can provide reassurance and understanding.

Taking care of your emotional well-being is crucial during pregnancy. Practicing self-care, engaging in activities that bring you joy and relaxation, and nurturing your relationships can help promote emotional balance. If you find that your emotions are overwhelming or affecting your daily life, don't hesitate to reach out to your healthcare provider or a mental health professional who can offer guidance and support.

Understanding the physical and emotional changes that occur during pregnancy is vital in navigating this transformative journey with confidence and grace. From the hormonal fluctuations that give rise to physical symptoms like breast tenderness, morning sickness, and fatigue, to the remarkable changes in your body shape and size, every aspect of pregnancy is a testament to the incredible process of nurturing new life.

By acknowledging and embracing these changes, you can develop a deeper appreciation for the marvel that is unfolding within you. Celebrate your body's ability to create and nurture a growing baby, and allow yourself to feel awe and wonder at the miracle of life.

Equally important is recognizing and addressing the emotional journey that accompanies pregnancy. The surge of hormones can impact your mood, leading to mood swings, heightened emotions, and occasional bouts of anxiety or depression. It's essential to give yourself permission to feel and process these emotions without judgment.

Engaging in self-care practices that nourish your emotional well-being is key. This may include engaging in relaxation techniques like meditation or deep breathing exercises, seeking support from your partner, family, or friends, and connecting with other expectant mothers who can relate to your experiences. Remember, you are not alone in this journey, and reaching out for support is a strength, not a weakness.

Throughout your pregnancy, regular prenatal check-ups with your healthcare provider will ensure that both your physical and emotional well-being are monitored. Don't hesitate to discuss any concerns or questions you may have during these appointments, as your healthcare team is there to support and guide you every step of the way.

As you navigate the physical and emotional changes of pregnancy, remember to be kind and gentle with yourself. Your body is doing something incredible, and it's natural to experience a range of feelings and sensations. Embrace the journey, nurture your well-being, and approach each day with gratitude and love for yourself and the life growing within you.

Embracing the Journey with Gratitude and Positivity

Pregnancy is a transformative journey that brings about immense changes, both physically and emotionally. Embracing this journey with gratitude and positivity can profoundly impact your experience, fostering a sense of joy, peace, and empowerment throughout the process.

Practicing Gratitude

Gratitude is a powerful tool that can shift your perspective and help you find joy in the little moments of pregnancy. Take a moment each day to reflect on the blessings and miracles unfolding within you. Express gratitude for the opportunity to carry and nurture a new life, for the support and love from your partner and loved ones, and for the incredible capabilities of your body. Keeping a gratitude journal or simply voicing your appreciation can cultivate a mindset of abundance and positivity.

Positive Affirmations

Affirmations are positive statements that you repeat to yourself, reinforcing beliefs and thoughts that uplift and empower you. During pregnancy, affirmations can serve as a reminder of your strength, resilience, and the love you have for yourself and your baby. Repeat affirmations that resonate with you, such as "I am capable of creating and nurturing life," "My body is strong and capable," or "I trust in the process of birth and motherhood." Let these affirmations become a source of inspiration and encouragement throughout your journey.

Fostering a Positive Mindset

Pregnancy, like any other life experience, presents its own set of challenges. However, approaching these challenges with a positive mindset can make a significant difference. Instead of focusing on the discomforts or uncertainties, shift your attention to the incredible journey of growth and creation. Surround yourself with positive influences, whether it's reading uplifting books, listening to inspiring podcasts, or connecting with other expectant mothers who radiate positivity. Cultivate an environment that nurtures optimism and supports your well-being.

Practicing Self-Care

Taking care of yourself physically, emotionally, and mentally is crucial for maintaining a positive outlook throughout your pregnancy. Engage in activities that bring you joy, relaxation, and peace. This can include gentle prenatal exercises, practicing prenatal yoga or meditation, indulging in nurturing baths, or enjoying a hobby that brings you happiness. Prioritize rest and relaxation, as well as adequate nutrition, to support your overall well-being. Remember, self-care is not selfish but a necessary investment in your own health and the health of your baby.

Finding Support

Surrounding yourself with a strong support system can provide the encouragement and positivity you need on your journey. Share your experiences, concerns, and joys with your partner, family, or close friends. Join prenatal classes or support groups where you can connect with other expectant mothers who are navigating a similar path. These connections can offer empathy, guidance, and a sense of community. By leaning on your support system, you create a space where positivity and encouragement can thrive.

Visualization and Bonding Rituals

Visualizing the birth you desire and creating bonding rituals with your baby can deepen your connection and nurture a positive mindset. Close your eyes and visualize a positive birth experience, envisioning yourself as confident, strong, and surrounded by love and support. Create special moments to bond with your baby, such as talking or singing to them, writing letters or creating a journal for them, or practicing gentle belly massage. These rituals foster a sense of connection and positivity, strengthening the bond between you and your baby.

Embracing the journey of pregnancy with gratitude and positivity is a transformative practice that allows you to fully experience the beauty and joy of this remarkable time. By cultivating gratitude, affirming your strengths, fostering a positive mindset, and practicing self-care, you create a nurturing environment for yourself and your growing baby.

Remember, every day is an opportunity to embrace the journey with an open heart and a positive outlook.

Chapter 2: Building Your Support Network

Pregnancy can be an overwhelming and emotional time. Building a strong support network can provide the guidance, empathy, and encouragement you need to navigate this transformative journey. Whether it's your partner, family, friends, or healthcare providers, your support system plays a crucial role in your physical and emotional well-being.

Communicating With Your Partner and Loved Ones

Effective communication with your partner and loved ones is essential during pregnancy. Sharing your experiences, concerns, and expectations can strengthen your relationships and provide the support you need throughout this transformative journey. Here are some tips for fostering open and meaningful communication:

1. Create a safe and non-judgmental space: Establish an environment where open and honest communication is welcomed. Ensure that all parties feel comfortable expressing their thoughts and emotions without fear of judgment or criticism. Encourage active listening, empathy, and understanding. By creating a safe space, you lay the foundation for deeper connections and mutual support.

2. Express your needs and expectations: Pregnancy can bring about a range of physical and emotional changes. Clearly communicate your needs, whether it's for physical comfort, emotional support, or assistance with household tasks. Help your partner and loved ones understand what you're going through by sharing your experiences and educating them about pregnancy. Remember, they may not fully

grasp the impact of pregnancy without your guidance.

3. Share your joys and concerns:
Celebrate the joys and milestones of your pregnancy together. Share the excitement of feeling the baby's movements, hearing their heartbeat, or seeing ultrasound images. Let your partner and loved ones be part of these memorable moments. Similarly, be open about your concerns, fears, and worries. Sharing your anxieties can help alleviate stress and allow your loved ones to offer reassurance and support.

4. Involve them in decision-making:
Include your partner and loved ones in the decision-making process related to your pregnancy and birth plan. Discuss options such as prenatal care, childbirth education classes, and birthing preferences. This involvement ensures that everyone feels included and has a voice in the decisions that impact your journey.

5. Attend prenatal appointments together:
Encourage your partner and loved ones to attend prenatal appointments with you. These visits offer an opportunity for them to witness the progress of your pregnancy, hear updates from healthcare providers, and ask any questions they may have. It also allows them to actively participate in your care and gain a deeper understanding of the journey you're undertaking.

6. Seek professional guidance if needed:
Sometimes, conversations with your partner or loved ones may become challenging or emotionally charged. In such cases, seeking the guidance of a professional, such as a couples counselor or therapist, can provide a neutral space for effective communication. A professional can help navigate difficult conversations, provide tools for active listening, and offer strategies to strengthen your relationships.

7. Be mindful of each other's experiences: Remember that pregnancy affects both you and your partner, albeit in different ways. Recognize and acknowledge their experiences, emotions, and concerns as well. Allow them to share their own journey and feelings. By fostering mutual understanding, empathy, and support, you can build a stronger bond as you embark on this transformative chapter together.

Effective communication with your partner and loved ones is vital during pregnancy. By creating a safe and open space, expressing your needs and expectations, sharing both joys and concerns, involving them in decision-making, attending prenatal appointments together, and seeking professional guidance if needed, you can build stronger connections and receive the support you need on this transformative journey. Remember, open communication is the key to nurturing and strengthening your relationships as you prepare to welcome your little one into the world.

Seeking Guidance From Healthcare Professionals

During pregnancy, healthcare professionals play a crucial role in ensuring the well-being of both you and your baby. Seeking guidance from these professionals can provide valuable information, support, and peace of mind throughout your journey. Here are some key aspects to consider when engaging with healthcare professionals:

1. Choosing the right healthcare provider: Selecting the right healthcare provider is essential for a positive and supportive pregnancy experience. Research different options, such as midwives, obstetricians, or family doctors, and consider their expertise, approach to care, and availability. Seek recommendations from trusted sources, and

schedule consultations to determine if their philosophy aligns with your preferences. Feeling comfortable and confident with your healthcare provider is vital for open communication and trust.

2. Attending regular prenatal appointments:
Prenatal appointments are essential for monitoring your health and the development of your baby. Regular check-ups allow healthcare professionals to track your progress, address any concerns, and provide necessary guidance. Attend these appointments consistently and use them as an opportunity to ask questions, discuss any physical or emotional changes you are experiencing, and seek clarification on prenatal care, nutrition, and exercise.

3. Communicating openly and honestly:
Be open and honest with your healthcare provider about your symptoms, concerns, and medical history. Clear and accurate communication helps them provide the best

possible care. Don't hesitate to share any emotional or mental health challenges you may be facing as well. Remember, healthcare professionals are there to support you and ensure your well-being, and they can only address your needs effectively if they are aware of them.

4. Asking questions and seeking information:
Take an active role in your prenatal care by asking questions and seeking information. This can help you understand the changes happening in your body, the progress of your pregnancy, and the options available to you. Ask about prenatal tests, potential complications, and the birthing process. Educating yourself empowers you to make informed decisions and actively participate in your care.

5. Discussing birth preferences and creating a birth plan:

Engage in open discussions with your healthcare provider about your birth preferences and create a birth plan together. Your birth plan outlines your desires for labor and delivery, including pain management options, birthing positions, and any specific requests you may have. Collaborating with your healthcare provider allows them to understand your preferences and work towards aligning your birth experience with your expectations as much as possible.

6. Seeking specialized care if needed:
In certain situations, specialized care may be required during pregnancy. Your healthcare provider will guide you if they identify any high-risk factors or if you have pre-existing medical conditions. In such cases, they may refer you to specialists such as maternal-fetal medicine experts or perinatologists. Seeking specialized care ensures that you receive the necessary

attention and expertise to manage any unique circumstances that arise.

7. Utilizing additional resources:
Healthcare professionals can provide a wealth of resources beyond medical care. They can recommend prenatal classes, support groups, or educational materials that can further enhance your knowledge and support network. Take advantage of these resources to connect with other expectant parents, learn about breastfeeding, newborn care, and parenting, and gain additional support throughout your pregnancy journey.

Seeking guidance from healthcare professionals is a fundamental aspect of a healthy and supported pregnancy. By choosing the right healthcare provider, attending regular prenatal appointments, communicating openly, asking questions, discussing birth preferences, seeking specialized care if needed, and utilizing additional resources, you can ensure that you receive the best possible care and support during this transformative time. Remember, your healthcare team is there to guide and empower you, making your journey toward motherhood as smooth and positive as possible.

Connecting with Other Expectant Mothers for Support and Friendship

Connecting with other expectant mothers can be a valuable source of support, friendship, and understanding during your pregnancy journey. Sharing experiences, seeking advice, and building relationships with women who are going through similar stages can provide a sense of community and camaraderie. Here are some ways to connect with other expectant mothers:

1. Prenatal classes and workshops:
Consider enrolling in prenatal classes and workshops offered in your community or

online. These classes not only provide valuable education on childbirth, breastfeeding, and newborn care but also create opportunities to connect with other expectant mothers. Sharing the same learning experiences can foster bonds and give you a network of women who can relate to your journey.

2. Joining support groups:
Look for local or online support groups specifically tailored for expectant mothers. These groups often provide a safe space to share experiences, concerns, and emotions. They can be an invaluable source of advice, empathy, and encouragement. Engaging with women who are going through similar challenges can help normalize your own experiences and provide a strong support network.

3. Participating in online forums and communities:

The internet offers a wealth of online forums and communities dedicated to pregnancy and motherhood. Joining these platforms allows you to connect with expectant mothers from around the world, enabling you to exchange stories, ask questions, and seek advice. Participate actively, contribute your own experiences, and engage with others to build lasting connections.

4. Attending local meet-ups or events:
Check for local meet-ups, baby fairs, or pregnancy-related events in your area. These gatherings provide an opportunity to meet other expectant mothers face-to-face and establish personal connections. Engage in conversations, exchange contact information, and arrange meet-ups outside of the organized events. Building friendships with women who live nearby can lead to lasting bonds and shared experiences as you embark on motherhood together.

5. Utilizing social media groups:

Social media platforms have become popular avenues for connecting with other expectant mothers. Join pregnancy-related groups or create your own closed group, inviting women from your social circle who are also expecting. These groups offer a convenient way to share updates, ask questions, and receive immediate support from a community of women who understand your journey.

6. Seeking out mom-to-be exercise classes or activities:
Participating in prenatal exercise classes, such as prenatal yoga, water aerobics, or dance, not only promotes physical well-being but also allows you to meet other expectant mothers with shared interests. Engaging in these activities together provides an opportunity to bond, support one another, and build friendships that can extend beyond pregnancy.

7. Reaching out to friends and acquaintances:
Don't forget to reach out to friends, acquaintances, or coworkers who have gone through pregnancy or recently become mothers. They can offer valuable insights, guidance, and support based on their own experiences. Sharing common connections can further strengthen your bond and create a support system within your existing social circle.

Remember, the journey of pregnancy is unique for every woman, but connecting with other expectant mothers can provide a sense of belonging and a shared understanding. By actively seeking out opportunities to connect, whether through classes, support groups, online communities, or personal connections, you can build a network of support and friendship that will continue to uplift you throughout your pregnancy and beyond.

Chapter 3: Nurturing Your Body

Taking care of your body is of utmost importance during pregnancy. As your body undergoes significant changes to accommodate the growth and development of your baby, it's essential to prioritize self-care and adopt healthy habits that support your well-being. Nurturing your body not only contributes to a healthier pregnancy but also lays the foundation for a smoother transition into motherhood. In this section, we will explore various ways to nourish and care for your body during this transformative time. From maintaining a balanced diet and staying hydrated to engaging in appropriate exercise and managing stress, we will delve into practical strategies that will help you navigate the physical and emotional changes of pregnancy with confidence and grace. By dedicating time and attention to nurturing your body, you are taking an active role in promoting your own health and ensuring the best possible start for your baby. So, let's embark on this journey of self-care and discover the power of nurturing your body during pregnancy.

Understanding the stages of pregnancy

Pregnancy is a remarkable journey that unfolds in stages, each marked by unique developments and milestones. Understanding these stages is key to navigating the physical and emotional changes you will experience throughout your pregnancy. In this section, we will explore the three main stages of pregnancy: the first trimester, the second trimester, and the third trimester. By gaining insight into each stage, you will be better equipped to embrace the transformations and make informed decisions about your health and well-being.

1. The First Trimester: Weeks 1-12
The first trimester is a time of excitement and adjustment as your body begins to prepare for pregnancy. During this stage, you may experience common symptoms such as morning sickness, fatigue, breast tenderness, and increased urination. Your baby undergoes rapid development, with major organs and body systems forming. This is also the period when you may have your first ultrasound, hear the baby's heartbeat, and share the news of your pregnancy with loved ones. It is crucial to prioritize your health during this stage, including taking prenatal vitamins, eating a balanced diet, and attending prenatal appointments.

2. The Second Trimester: Weeks 13-27
The second trimester is often considered the most enjoyable stage of pregnancy. Many women experience relief from early pregnancy symptoms, and a newfound

energy may accompany this period. Your baby's growth accelerates during this time, and you may begin to feel their movements, a milestone that deepens the connection between you and your little one. It's important to continue practicing self-care, engaging in regular exercise, and eating nutritious meals. You will also have regular check-ups with your healthcare provider to monitor your baby's growth and well-being.

3. The Third Trimester: Weeks 28-40

The third trimester brings you closer to the anticipation of meeting your baby. However, this stage can also present unique challenges as your body continues to adapt to accommodate your growing baby. You may experience discomfort, such as backaches, swelling, and difficulty sleeping. It's important to prioritize rest, practice relaxation techniques, and seek support from your healthcare provider for managing any discomfort. As you approach your due date, you will have more frequent prenatal visits to monitor your baby's position, prepare for labor and delivery, and discuss your birth plan.

Understanding the stages of pregnancy allows you to anticipate the changes you will experience physically and emotionally, empowering you to make informed decisions about your care and well-being. Each stage presents its own joys and challenges, and by embracing the journey with knowledge and preparation, you can navigate pregnancy with confidence and ease.

Maintaining a healthy diet and exercise routine

A healthy diet and regular exercise are essential components of a well-rounded pregnancy routine. Nourishing your body with the right foods and staying physically active can promote your overall well-being, support your baby's development, and prepare your body for childbirth. In this section, we will delve into the importance of maintaining a healthy diet and exercise routine throughout your pregnancy, providing practical tips and guidelines to help you make informed choices for you and your baby.

Nourishing Your Body with a Healthy Diet

During pregnancy, your body requires additional nutrients to support the growth and development of your baby. A well-balanced diet rich in essential vitamins, minerals, proteins, and healthy fats is crucial for your overall health and the healthy development of your baby. Here are some key considerations for maintaining a healthy diet during pregnancy:

1. Focus on nutrient-dense foods:
Choose whole, unprocessed foods that are packed with essential nutrients. Include a

variety of fruits, vegetables, whole grains, lean proteins, and healthy fats in your meals. These foods provide the vitamins, minerals, and fiber necessary for both you and your baby's well-being.

2. Prioritize hydration:
Drink plenty of water throughout the day to stay hydrated. Aim for at least eight to ten glasses of water daily, and adjust your intake as needed based on your activity level and the weather. Staying hydrated can help prevent constipation, reduce swelling, and support your body's various functions.

3. Ensure adequate protein intake:
Protein is essential for the growth and repair of tissues in both you and your baby. Include lean meats, poultry, fish, eggs, legumes, nuts, and dairy products in your diet to meet your protein needs. If you follow a vegetarian or vegan diet, ensure you're getting adequate protein from plant-based

sources such as tofu, tempeh, lentils, and quinoa.

4. Incorporate plenty of fruits and vegetables:
Fruits and vegetables provide a wide array of vitamins, minerals, and antioxidants. Aim to include a variety of colors in your diet to ensure you're receiving a broad range of nutrients. Fresh or frozen options are both excellent choices, but be cautious with unwashed produce to minimize the risk of foodborne illnesses.

5. Consume sufficient calcium and iron:
Calcium is essential for your baby's bone development, while iron supports the production of red blood cells. Incorporate calcium-rich foods such as dairy products, leafy greens, and fortified plant-based milk alternatives. Increase your iron intake through sources like lean meats, beans, spinach, and fortified cereals. Consult with

your healthcare provider about the need for additional iron or calcium supplements.

6. Practice mindful eating:
Pay attention to your hunger and fullness cues, and practice mindful eating. Eat slowly, savoring each bite, and stop when you feel comfortably satisfied. This helps prevent overeating and promotes better digestion.

7. Limit certain foods and substances:
Some foods and substances should be avoided or limited during pregnancy. These include raw or undercooked meat, fish high in mercury, unpasteurized dairy products, raw or undercooked eggs, excessive caffeine, alcohol, and tobacco. Consult your healthcare provider for specific guidelines and recommendations.

Engaging in Safe and Beneficial Exercise

Regular exercise during pregnancy offers numerous benefits, including improved cardiovascular health, increased energy levels, better mood regulation, and enhanced strength and stamina for childbirth. However, it's essential to choose exercises that are safe and appropriate for each stage of pregnancy. Here are some guidelines for incorporating exercise into your pregnancy routine:

1. Consult with your healthcare provider:
Before starting or continuing an exercise routine during pregnancy, consult with your healthcare provider. They can evaluate your health and provide specific recommendations based on your individual circumstances.

2. Choose low-impact activities:
Opt for low-impact exercises that are gentle on your joints and minimize the risk of injury. Walking, swimming, prenatal yoga, stationary cycling, and water aerobics are

excellent options. These activities help improve cardiovascular fitness, strengthen muscles, and maintain flexibility.

3. Warm up and cool down:
Always begin your exercise session with a warm-up to prepare your body for physical activity. Gentle stretches and movements increase blood flow to your muscles and reduce the risk of injury. After your workout, take time to cool down and stretch to promote muscle recovery and flexibility.

4. Listen to your body:
Pay attention to your body's signals during exercise. If you experience pain, dizziness, shortness of breath, or any other discomfort, stop exercising and consult your healthcare provider. Modify or adapt exercises as needed to accommodate your changing body.

5. Stay hydrated and avoid overheating:

Drink plenty of water before, during, and after your workout to stay hydrated. Avoid exercising in hot and humid environments to prevent overheating, as it can be dangerous for both you and your baby.

6. Use proper form and technique:
Maintain good posture and use proper form and technique during exercises to avoid strain or injury. If you are unsure about the correct technique, consider working with a certified prenatal fitness instructor who can guide you.

7. Modify as your pregnancy progresses:
As your pregnancy advances, your body's capabilities and comfort levels may change. Modify exercises accordingly to accommodate your growing belly and any physical limitations. Avoid activities that involve lying flat on your back, as this can restrict blood flow to your baby.

8. Incorporate pelvic floor exercises:

Strengthening your pelvic floor muscles through Kegel exercises can be beneficial during pregnancy and postpartum. These exercises help support your pelvic organs, reduce the risk of urinary incontinence, and aid in postpartum recovery.

9. Practice relaxation and breathing techniques:
Incorporate relaxation techniques and deep breathing exercises into your exercise routine. These techniques help reduce stress, promote relaxation, and can be beneficial during labor and delivery.

Remember, every pregnancy is unique, and it's crucial to listen to your body and work within your comfort levels. If you have any concerns or medical conditions, consult your healthcare provider for personalized advice and exercise recommendations. By maintaining a healthy diet and engaging in safe and beneficial exercise, you can support your overall well-being and contribute to a healthier and more comfortable pregnancy experience.

Managing Common Discomforts and Promoting Self-Care

Pregnancy is a transformative journey that brings about incredible joy and anticipation. However, it also comes with its fair share of common discomforts. From nausea and fatigue to backaches and swelling, it's important to equip yourself with strategies to manage these discomforts and prioritize self-care. In this section, we will explore various techniques and practices to help you navigate the challenges of pregnancy and promote your overall well-being.

Nausea and Morning Sickness

Nausea and morning sickness are common discomforts experienced during pregnancy, particularly in the first trimester. To manage these symptoms, consider the following:

1. Eat small, frequent meals:
Instead of consuming large meals, opt for smaller, more frequent meals throughout the day. This can help prevent your stomach from becoming too empty or too full, which can trigger nausea.

2. Avoid triggers:
Identify any specific foods, smells, or situations that trigger your nausea and try to avoid them. This may include spicy or greasy foods, strong odors, or certain environments.

3. Stay hydrated:
Sip on fluids throughout the day to stay hydrated, as dehydration can worsen nausea. Try drinking cold or carbonated beverages, ginger ale, or sucking on ice chips to ease symptoms.

4. Ginger:

Ginger has natural anti-nausea properties. Consider consuming ginger tea, ginger candies, or adding fresh ginger to your meals to help alleviate nausea.

Fatigue and Low Energy

Pregnancy can often leave you feeling fatigued and low on energy. To manage these symptoms, try the following:

1. Prioritize rest and sleep:
Listen to your body's signals and make sleep a priority. Aim for seven to eight hours of quality sleep each night, and consider taking short naps during the day to recharge.

2. Practice relaxation techniques:
Incorporate relaxation techniques, such as deep breathing exercises, meditation, or prenatal yoga, into your daily routine. These practices can help reduce stress, improve sleep quality, and boost your energy levels.

3. Engage in gentle exercise:
While it may seem counterintuitive, engaging in regular, gentle exercise can actually help alleviate fatigue and boost energy levels. Incorporate activities like walking, swimming, or prenatal yoga into your routine. Consult with your healthcare provider for exercise recommendations that suit your individual circumstances.

Backaches and Body Discomfort

As your baby grows, you may experience backaches and overall body discomfort. Consider these strategies to manage these discomforts:

1. Maintain good posture:
Practice good posture to alleviate strain on your back and body. Avoid slouching and try to distribute your body weight evenly.

2. Use proper body mechanics:

When lifting objects or performing daily tasks, use proper body mechanics to minimize strain on your back. Bend from your knees, not your waist, and avoid twisting motions.

3. Wear supportive footwear:
Opt for comfortable and supportive shoes to provide proper cushioning and alignment for your feet and back. Avoid high heels, as they can exacerbate backaches.

4. Use heat or cold therapy:
Apply a heating pad or take a warm bath to soothe back aches and relax tense muscles. Alternatively, use a cold pack or ice wrapped in a thin towel to reduce inflammation and numb the area.

Swelling and Fluid Retention

Swelling, particularly in the legs, ankles, and feet, is a common discomfort during pregnancy. To manage swelling and fluid retention, try the following:

1. Stay active:
Engaging in regular, low-impact exercise, such as walking or swimming, can help improve circulation and reduce swelling. Avoid prolonged periods of sitting or standing in one position.

2. Elevate your legs:
Elevate your legs whenever possible to reduce swelling. Prop your feet up on a pillow or ottoman while sitting or lying down to help improve circulation and encourage fluid drainage.

3. Wear comfortable clothing and footwear:
Opt for loose-fitting, comfortable clothing that doesn't constrict your circulation. Choose supportive shoes that provide adequate cushioning and avoid tight socks or stockings that can restrict blood flow.

4. Stay hydrated:
Drinking plenty of water throughout the day can help flush out excess fluids from your body and reduce swelling. Aim to drink at least eight to ten glasses of water daily, or as recommended by your healthcare provider.

5. Avoid excessive sodium intake:
High sodium intake can contribute to fluid retention. Limit your consumption of processed foods, fast food, and salty snacks. Instead, opt for fresh, whole foods that are naturally low in sodium.

Promoting Self-Care

Taking care of yourself is essential during pregnancy. Here are some self-care practices to prioritize:

1. Practice relaxation techniques:
Engage in activities that promote relaxation and reduce stress. This may include deep

breathing exercises, meditation, gentle stretching, or taking soothing baths. Find what works best for you and incorporate it into your daily routine.

2. Pamper yourself:
Indulge in self-care activities that make you feel good. This could be treating yourself to a prenatal massage, getting a manicure or pedicure, or simply taking time to read a book or watch your favorite movie.

3. Stay connected with loved ones:
Maintain strong connections with your partner, family, and friends. Share your feelings and concerns, and seek support when needed. Surround yourself with positive and understanding individuals who can provide encouragement and reassurance.

4. Seek emotional support:
Pregnancy can bring about a range of emotions. If you find yourself feeling

overwhelmed, anxious, or experiencing mood swings, consider seeking emotional support from a therapist, counselor, or support group. Talking to a professional can help you navigate these emotions and provide valuable coping strategies.

5. Prioritize your needs:
Remember to prioritize your own needs and well-being. Practice saying no when necessary, delegate tasks to others, and give yourself permission to rest and take breaks when needed. Taking care of yourself allows you to better care for your growing baby.

By implementing these strategies and prioritizing self-care, you can effectively manage common discomforts and promote your overall well-being during pregnancy. Each woman's pregnancy journey is unique, so it's important to listen to your body, consult with your healthcare provider, and adapt these suggestions to suit your individual circumstances. Embrace the opportunity to care for yourself, as it contributes to a positive and fulfilling pregnancy experience.

Chapter 4: Cultivating Emotional Well-being

Pregnancy is a time of incredible joy, anticipation, and transformation. As you prepare to welcome a new life into the world, it's important to recognize and prioritize your emotional well-being. Pregnancy can bring about a range of emotions, from excitement and happiness to anxiety and vulnerability. Cultivating emotional well-being during this transformative journey is crucial not only for your own mental health but also for the overall well-being of you and your baby.

In this chapter, we will explore the importance of nurturing your emotional well-being throughout pregnancy and provide practical strategies and techniques to help you navigate the emotional roller coaster that often accompanies this extraordinary time in your life. By taking proactive steps to care for your emotional health, you can enhance your pregnancy experience, foster positive connections with your baby, and build a solid foundation for the transition into motherhood.

Coping with Hormonal Changes and Mood Swings

Pregnancy brings about significant hormonal changes that can have a profound impact on your emotional well-being. Hormones such as estrogen, progesterone, and human chorionic gonadotropin (hCG) fluctuate throughout pregnancy, leading to mood swings and emotional ups and downs. Coping with these hormonal changes is an essential part of maintaining your emotional well-being during pregnancy. In this section, we will explore practical strategies to help you navigate hormonal fluctuations and manage mood swings effectively.

1. Recognize the role of hormones:

Understanding that hormonal changes are a natural part of pregnancy can help you gain perspective and normalize your emotional experiences. Remind yourself that these fluctuations are temporary and a normal aspect of the pregnancy journey.

2. Communicate with your partner:
Open and honest communication with your partner is crucial during this time. Let them know about the hormonal changes you are experiencing and how they may affect your emotions. Together, you can find ways to support each other and navigate through any challenges that arise.

3. Practice self-care:
Engaging in self-care activities can help alleviate mood swings and promote emotional well-being. Take time for yourself each day to do something that brings you joy and relaxation. This can include activities like taking a warm bath, practicing

mindfulness or meditation, indulging in a hobby, or spending time in nature.

4. Get regular exercise:
Physical activity has been shown to positively impact mood and reduce stress. Engage in regular exercise that is safe and suitable for your pregnancy. This can include walking, swimming, prenatal yoga, or low-impact aerobics. Consult with your healthcare provider for exercise recommendations tailored to your specific needs.

5. Seek support from other expectant mothers:
Connecting with other pregnant women who are going through similar experiences can provide a sense of validation and support. Joining prenatal support groups or online communities can offer a safe space to share your emotions, seek advice, and gain insights from others who understand what you are going through.

6. Practice stress management techniques:
Stress can exacerbate mood swings and make it more challenging to cope with hormonal changes. Implement stress management techniques such as deep breathing exercises, progressive muscle relaxation, or engaging in activities that help you unwind and relax. Consider incorporating practices like prenatal yoga, meditation, or guided imagery into your routine.

7. Prioritize sleep:
Adequate rest and sleep are crucial for emotional well-being. Create a sleep-friendly environment, establish a regular bedtime routine, and ensure you have a comfortable sleep space. If discomfort or pregnancy-related issues interfere with your sleep, speak with your healthcare provider for guidance on improving your sleep quality.

8. Maintain a balanced diet:
A well-balanced diet can have a positive impact on mood and energy levels. Opt for nutritious foods that support hormonal balance and provide essential nutrients. Include plenty of fruits, vegetables, whole grains, lean proteins, and healthy fats in your meals. Stay hydrated by drinking enough water throughout the day.

9. Seek professional help when needed:
If mood swings become overwhelming or significantly impact your daily functioning, don't hesitate to reach out to a healthcare professional. They can provide guidance, support, and, if necessary, recommend appropriate interventions or therapies to help you navigate through these challenges.

Remember, mood swings and hormonal changes are common during pregnancy, but there are strategies and support available to help you cope effectively. By implementing these techniques and seeking support when needed, you can navigate through these emotional fluctuations with greater ease, promoting a more positive and balanced emotional well-being throughout your pregnancy journey.

Addressing Fears and Anxieties

Pregnancy is often accompanied by fears and anxieties, ranging from concerns about the health of your baby to worries about the birthing process and becoming a parent. Addressing these fears and anxieties is crucial for your emotional well-being during pregnancy. In this section, we will explore practical strategies to help you identify, understand, and address your fears and anxieties effectively.

1. Acknowledge and express your fears:
Start by acknowledging and accepting your fears. It's normal to experience a wide range of emotions during pregnancy, including fear and anxiety. Give yourself permission to

express your concerns and emotions without judgment.

2. Educate yourself:
Knowledge is empowering. Educate yourself about pregnancy, childbirth, and parenting. Attend prenatal classes, read books, and consult reliable sources of information. Understanding the process and having accurate information can help alleviate fears and provide a sense of control.

3. Openly communicate with your partner:
Share your fears and anxieties with your partner. Open and honest communication can provide comfort and support. Discuss your concerns, listen to each other's perspectives, and explore ways to address those fears together.

4. Seek reassurance from healthcare professionals:
Your healthcare team is there to support you and address any concerns you may have.

Schedule regular prenatal appointments and use these opportunities to ask questions, share your fears, and seek reassurance. Trust in the expertise and guidance of your healthcare provider.

5. Connect with other expectant parents:
Joining support groups or connecting with other expectant parents can help normalize your fears and provide a sense of community. Sharing experiences, exchanging advice, and hearing others' stories can offer comfort and reassurance.

6. Practice relaxation techniques:
Engaging in relaxation techniques can help alleviate anxiety and promote emotional well-being. Explore techniques such as deep breathing exercises, guided imagery, meditation, or prenatal yoga. Find what resonates with you and incorporate these practices into your daily routine.

7. Challenge negative thoughts:

Often, fears and anxieties stem from negative thoughts and assumptions. Challenge these thoughts by questioning their validity and replacing them with more positive and realistic ones. Use affirmations or mantras to counteract negative thinking patterns.

8. Create a birth plan:
If concerns about the birthing process are causing anxiety, consider creating a birth plan. A birth plan outlines your preferences and helps you feel more prepared and in control. Discuss your options with your healthcare provider, attend childbirth education classes, and seek information to make informed decisions.

9. Practice self-care and stress management:
Taking care of your physical and emotional well-being is crucial in addressing fears and anxieties. Prioritize self-care activities that promote relaxation and reduce stress. This

can include activities like taking baths, practicing mindfulness, engaging in hobbies, or spending time in nature.

10. Seek professional help if needed:
If fears and anxieties become overwhelming and significantly impact your daily life, seeking professional help is important. A therapist or counselor experienced in pregnancy-related issues can provide guidance, support, and strategies to manage and overcome your fears and anxieties.

Remember, it is natural to have fears and anxieties during pregnancy. By addressing them proactively and seeking support, you can navigate through these emotions with greater ease. Each person's journey is unique, and it's essential to be patient and compassionate with yourself as you work through your fears and anxieties. Trust in your own resilience and the support available to you, and believe in your ability to navigate this transformative journey with strength and courage.

Practicing Mindfulness and Relaxation Techniques

Practicing mindfulness and relaxation techniques during pregnancy can significantly contribute to your emotional well-being. These practices help you stay present, manage stress, and cultivate a sense of calm amidst the many changes and challenges of pregnancy. In this section, we will explore various mindfulness and relaxation techniques that you can incorporate into your daily routine to promote a sense of peace and emotional balance.

1. Deep Breathing Exercises:
Deep breathing exercises are simple yet powerful techniques that can instantly calm your mind and relax your body. Find a quiet and comfortable space, close your eyes,

and take slow, deep breaths. Inhale deeply through your nose, allowing your abdomen to expand, and exhale slowly through your mouth, releasing any tension or stress with each breath. Practice this deep breathing exercise for a few minutes whenever you feel overwhelmed or anxious.

2. Guided Imagery and Visualization:
Guided imagery and visualization involve creating mental images or scenarios that promote relaxation and positive emotions. Find a quiet space, close your eyes, and imagine yourself in a peaceful and serene environment. Visualize the sights, sounds, and sensations of this calming place, allowing yourself to fully immerse in the experience. You can also use guided imagery recordings or apps specifically designed for pregnancy to enhance relaxation and connect with your baby.

3. Progressive Muscle Relaxation:

Progressive muscle relaxation is a technique that involves systematically tensing and releasing different muscle groups to promote relaxation and release physical tension. Start by sitting or lying down in a comfortable position. Begin with your toes and gradually work your way up through your legs, abdomen, chest, arms, and neck, tensing and then releasing each muscle group. Pay attention to the sensation of relaxation as you release the tension. This practice can help alleviate muscle tension and promote a state of deep relaxation.

4. Mindful Eating:
Pregnancy is an excellent time to practice mindful eating, which involves bringing awareness and attention to your food choices, eating habits, and physical sensations while eating. Before eating, take a moment to pause and express gratitude for the nourishment your meal provides. Slow down your eating pace, savor each

bite, and pay attention to the flavors, textures, and sensations. This practice helps you develop a healthier relationship with food, enhances digestion, and promotes overall well-being.

5. Prenatal Yoga and Stretching:
Prenatal yoga and gentle stretching exercises can promote relaxation, flexibility, and body awareness. Attend prenatal yoga classes specifically designed for pregnant women or follow along with online videos or apps. These practices incorporate breathing techniques, gentle stretches, and poses that help release tension, improve circulation, and promote relaxation. Always consult with your healthcare provider before engaging in any physical activity during pregnancy.

6. Mindful Walking:
Engaging in mindful walking allows you to connect with nature, practice present-moment awareness, and experience the physical sensations of

movement. Find a peaceful outdoor setting, such as a park or nature trail, and start walking at a comfortable pace. Focus your attention on the sensation of your feet touching the ground, the rhythm of your breath, and the sights and sounds around you. Be fully present in the experience, observing without judgment.

7. Meditation and Mindfulness Practices:
Meditation is a powerful tool for cultivating mindfulness and promoting emotional well-being. Set aside dedicated time each day to sit in a quiet space, close your eyes, and focus your attention on your breath, a mantra, or a specific point of focus. As thoughts arise, gently acknowledge them without judgment and return your focus to your breath or chosen point of focus. You can also explore mindfulness practices in daily activities such as mindful dishwashing, mindful showering, or mindful parenting moments.

8. Sensory Relaxation Techniques:
Engaging your senses can enhance relaxation and promote mindfulness. Here are some sensory relaxation techniques you can try:

- Aromatherapy: Use essential oils known for their calming properties, such as lavender or chamomile. You can use a diffuser, add a few drops to a warm bath, or create a soothing massage oil.

- Music and Sound Therapy: Listen to calming music or nature sounds that help you relax. You can create a playlist of gentle and soothing melodies or use apps that offer guided meditation or relaxation music specifically designed for pregnancy.

- Warm Compresses: Place a warm compress or heating pad on areas of tension, such as your shoulders or lower back. The warmth can help soothe muscles and promote relaxation.

- Mindful Touch: Engage in self-massage or ask your partner to give you a gentle massage. Focus on the sensations of touch, allowing yourself to relax and release tension in your body.

- Visual Relaxation: Create a calming visual environment by surrounding yourself with objects or images that evoke a sense of peace and tranquility. This can include soft lighting, nature-inspired artwork, or candles.

Remember, incorporating these mindfulness and relaxation techniques into your daily routine requires consistency and practice. Find what resonates with you and adapt them to your preferences and needs. Embrace the opportunity to connect with your body, nurture your emotional well-being, and bond with your baby as you navigate the transformative journey of pregnancy.

Chapter 5: Creating a Safe and Nurturing Environment

Creating a safe and nurturing environment is vital during pregnancy as it supports your well-being, promotes a sense of security, and fosters a positive experience for both you and your growing baby. Your surroundings can significantly impact your emotional and physical health, as well as your overall pregnancy journey. In this chapter, we will explore strategies to help you create a safe and nurturing environment that supports your needs and enhances your pregnancy experience.

Preparing Your Home for the Baby's Arrival

Preparing your home for the arrival of your baby is an exciting and important step in creating a safe and nurturing environment. It involves making necessary adjustments, organizing essential items, and ensuring that your home is ready to welcome your little one. In this section, we will explore in detail how you can prepare your home for the baby's arrival, covering key areas such as the nursery, safety measures, and practical considerations.

1. Designing the Nursery:
The nursery is where your baby will spend a significant amount of time, so it's important to create a comfortable and functional space. Start by choosing a suitable room that can be easily accessed and has good ventilation. Consider the following aspects:

- Painting and Decor: Choose soothing and non-toxic paint colors for the walls. Opt for a theme or design that creates a calming and joyful atmosphere. Decorate with wall art, mobiles, and soft furnishings that are safe and age-appropriate.

- Furniture: Invest in essential furniture items such as a crib, changing table, dresser, and comfortable chair for feeding and bonding. Ensure that all furniture meets safety standards, has rounded edges, and is securely assembled.

- Storage: Install storage solutions such as shelves, baskets, and drawers to organize baby essentials like diapers, clothing, blankets, and toys. Keep frequently used items easily accessible.

- Lighting: Consider installing blackout curtains or shades to create a sleep-friendly environment. Place soft, adjustable lighting options such as nightlights or dimmers for nighttime feeding and diaper changes.

2. Ensuring Safety:
Creating a safe environment is paramount when preparing for your baby's arrival. Take the following measures to ensure their safety:

- Childproofing: Baby-proof your home by securing cabinets, blocking off staircases, and installing outlet covers and safety gates. Eliminate potential hazards such as loose cords, small objects, and sharp edges.

- Smoke and Carbon Monoxide Detectors: Install smoke and carbon monoxide detectors on each floor of your home, especially near sleeping areas.

- Fire Safety: Familiarize yourself with fire safety protocols and have fire extinguishers readily available. Create an escape plan and ensure that all family members are aware of it.

- Baby Monitor: Invest in a reliable baby monitor to keep a watchful eye on your little one, especially during sleep times.

- Crib Safety: Ensure that the crib meets safety standards, with a firm mattress and fitted sheet. Remove any soft bedding, pillows, or stuffed animals that pose a suffocation risk.

3. Practical Considerations:
Preparing your home goes beyond safety measures. It's essential to think about practical aspects that will make caring for your baby easier:

- Diaper Changing Area: Set up a dedicated diaper changing station in the nursery or a convenient area of your home. Stock it with diapers, wipes, diaper rash cream, and a diaper pail.

- Feeding Area: If you plan to breastfeed, create a cozy and comfortable nursing area with a nursing chair or a comfortable spot with pillows for support. If you're bottle-feeding, organize bottles, sterilizers, and formula supplies.

- Baby Care Essentials: Gather essential items such as baby clothes, swaddles, blankets, burp cloths, towels, and bathing supplies. Organize them for easy access in drawers or storage bins.

- Laundry and Cleaning: Prepare a designated space for baby laundry, including a hamper, detergent suitable for baby clothes, and a drying rack. Ensure that cleaning products used in your home are baby-safe.

- Stocking Up: Start gradually stocking up on baby essentials such as diapers, wipes, baby toiletries, and feeding supplies. Consider having a supply of essentials on hand for the first few weeks after the baby's arrival.

As you prepare your home for the baby's arrival, remember that it's an ongoing process that can be done gradually over time. Don't feel overwhelmed by trying to accomplish everything at once. Take it step by step, focusing on one area or task at a time. Involve your partner, family members, or friends in the process to make it more enjoyable and efficient.

Additionally, consider involving a professional home safety inspector or a babyproofing expert to assess your home and provide guidance on potential safety hazards you may have overlooked. They can offer valuable insights and recommendations specific to your home's layout and your baby's needs.

In the weeks leading up to your due date, it's also a good idea to pack a hospital bag with essentials for both you and the baby. This way, you'll be prepared when the time comes to head to the hospital.

Remember that as you prepare your home, it's essential to balance functionality with creating a warm and inviting space for your baby. Your home should be a place of love, comfort, and security. Take time to infuse personal touches that reflect your family's personality and values.

Lastly, don't forget to take care of yourself during this process. Pregnancy can be physically demanding, so listen to your body and take breaks when needed. Pace yourself and ask for help if necessary. This time of preparation should be a joyous and exciting experience as you anticipate the arrival of your little one.

By taking the time to prepare your home for the baby's arrival, you are creating an environment that nurtures their growth, development, and well-being. It provides a foundation of safety and support that will allow you to focus on bonding with your baby and enjoying the precious moments of early parenthood.

Chapter 6: Bonding with Your Baby

The bond between a mother and her baby is one of the most profound and magical connections in the world. It begins during pregnancy and continues to grow and evolve as your baby enters the world. Bonding is a vital process that not only strengthens the emotional attachment between you and your baby but also promotes their overall development and well-being. In this section, we will explore the importance of bonding, various ways to foster this connection, and the benefits it brings to both you and your little one.

The bond you establish with your baby sets the foundation for their future relationships, social interactions, and emotional well-being. It is a unique and beautiful journey that starts long before you hold your baby in your arms. Throughout pregnancy, you have the opportunity to begin building a deep and loving connection as you nurture your baby in the womb. After birth, the bond continues to grow through moments of physical closeness, eye contact, gentle touch, and responsive care.

In this section, we will delve into the significance of bonding with your baby and offer practical guidance on how to enhance this special relationship. We will explore techniques that promote bonding during pregnancy, as well as ways to strengthen the bond after birth. From the first fluttering kicks to the precious moments of skin-to-skin contact and beyond, every interaction contributes to the bond you share with your baby.

Connecting with Your Growing Baby

Connecting with your growing baby is a precious and transformative experience that begins during pregnancy. As your baby develops and grows within the womb, there are numerous ways to establish a deep and meaningful connection. These moments of connection not only strengthen the bond between you and your baby but also provide a sense of joy, comfort, and anticipation as you eagerly await their arrival. In this section, we will explore in detail how you can connect with your growing baby during pregnancy.

1. Talking and Singing to Your Baby:
Your voice is one of the most powerful tools to connect with your baby. Engage in regular conversations, read aloud, or sing songs to your baby. Your soothing voice and familiar rhythms create a sense of comfort and security for them. As you talk or sing, place your hands on your belly, feeling the gentle movements and imagining the

connection you're forging with your little one.

2. Gentle Touch and Massage:
Touch is a powerful means of communication and connection. Place your hands on your belly and gently caress or massage the area. You can use natural oils or lotions to enhance the experience. Pay attention to your baby's movements and respond to their kicks and wiggles with gentle touches or light pressure. This physical connection allows both you and your baby to experience a sense of closeness and reassurance.

3. Mindful Belly Bonding:
Set aside dedicated time each day to connect with your baby in a calm and mindful way. Find a comfortable position, close your eyes, and focus on your breathing. Visualize your baby within the womb, sending them love, and positive energy. Imagine the bond between you and

your baby growing stronger with each breath. This practice not only fosters a sense of connection but also helps you relax and reduce stress.

4. Playing Music:
Play soothing and uplifting music for your baby. Choose a variety of genres and notice how your baby responds to different types of music. You can experiment with classical music, gentle lullabies, or even play songs that hold a special meaning to you. Pay attention to your baby's movements and reactions, as they may respond to the sound and rhythm.

5. Engaging in Gentle Movements:
Physical activity can also be a way to connect with your baby. Engage in gentle exercises like prenatal yoga or take leisurely walks while focusing your attention on the sensations within your body. Notice your baby's movements as you move, imagining

them experiencing the same sense of motion and rhythm.

6. Creating a Pregnancy Journal:
Keep a journal to document your thoughts, feelings, and experiences throughout your pregnancy. Write letters to your baby, expressing your hopes, dreams, and love. This journal becomes a treasured keepsake that you can share with your child as they grow older, deepening the connection and providing a glimpse into the beautiful journey of their beginnings.

Remember, connecting with your growing baby is a personal and unique experience. Follow your intuition and embrace the activities that resonate with you and your baby. Each interaction is an opportunity to strengthen the bond and lay the foundation for a lifelong connection. As you connect with your growing baby, allow yourself to be fully present, savoring each moment, and cherishing the incredible miracle of life unfolding within you.

The Art of Pregnancy Fashion

Pregnancy is a remarkable journey filled with joy, anticipation, and countless changes. As your body goes through the beautiful transformation of nurturing a new life, your sense of style can also evolve to embrace and celebrate your changing figure. Pregnancy fashion is an art form that allows you to express your individuality, showcase your unique style, and feel confident and beautiful during this special time. In this section, we will explore the art of pregnancy fashion, offering tips, inspiration, and guidance to help you curate a stylish and comfortable wardrobe that embraces your pregnancy glow.

Gone are the days when pregnancy fashion was limited to oversized and shapeless clothing. Today, there is a plethora of stylish options designed specifically for expectant mothers. From chic maternity dresses and trendy tops to versatile bottoms and comfortable loungewear, the world of pregnancy fashion offers a wide range of choices to suit every taste and occasion.

The art of pregnancy fashion goes beyond simply finding clothes that fit. It involves embracing your changing body, accentuating your best features, and adapting your personal style to accommodate your growing belly. It's about feeling empowered, confident, and comfortable in your own skin as you navigate this unique phase of life.

In this section, we will delve into the world of pregnancy fashion, exploring various aspects that contribute to creating a stylish and functional maternity wardrobe.

Dressing Stylishly and Comfortably

Dressing stylishly and comfortably during pregnancy is an art that allows you to embrace your changing body while expressing your unique sense of style. It's essential to choose clothing that not only looks fashionable but also prioritizes your comfort and well-being. With a few key considerations, you can curate a maternity wardrobe that effortlessly combines style and comfort. Here are some detailed tips for dressing stylishly and comfortably during pregnancy:

1. Prioritize Fit and Function: As your body undergoes changes during pregnancy, it's crucial to choose clothing that provides a comfortable and flattering fit. Opt for maternity-specific clothing that is designed to accommodate your growing belly. Look for styles with stretchy fabrics, adjustable waistbands, and strategic gathering or ruching that allows the clothes to adapt to your changing shape. Maternity jeans, leggings, and dresses with empire

waistlines are popular choices that offer both style and comfort.

2. Choose Breathable Fabrics: Pregnancy can bring about changes in body temperature and increased perspiration. To stay comfortable, select clothing made from breathable fabrics such as cotton, linen, and bamboo. These materials allow air circulation, keeping you cool and preventing discomfort. Avoid synthetic fabrics that can trap heat and moisture against your skin.

3. Opt for Layering: Layering is an excellent technique for creating stylish and adaptable outfits during pregnancy. Choose lightweight, layer-friendly pieces like cardigans, blazers, and vests. Layering not only adds dimension to your outfit but also allows you to adjust your clothing according to your comfort level and changing weather conditions.

4. Embrace Empire Waistlines and A-Line Silhouettes: Empire waistlines and A-line silhouettes are flattering and comfortable choices for pregnancy fashion. These styles emphasize your bustline and flow loosely over your growing belly, providing ample room for movement and growth. Empire waist dresses, tunics, and tops are versatile options that can be dressed up or down for various occasions.

5. Play with Prints and Colors: Incorporating prints and colors into your maternity wardrobe can add a vibrant touch to your outfits and boost your mood. Opt for prints like stripes, florals, or geometric patterns that flatter your body shape. Experiment with different color palettes to find shades that complement your skin tone and make you feel confident and radiant.

6. Don't Neglect Footwear: As your pregnancy progresses, you may experience swelling and changes in shoe size. Opt for

comfortable footwear options that provide adequate support and cushioning for your feet. Choose shoes with low or moderate heels to prevent discomfort and reduce the risk of falls. Consider slip-on styles or shoes with adjustable closures to accommodate any swelling.

7. Invest in Maternity Undergarments: Maternity undergarments, including bras and underwear, are specifically designed to provide comfort and support during pregnancy. As your breasts and body change, it's essential to invest in properly fitting undergarments that offer sufficient support and minimize discomfort. Look for bras with adjustable straps and expandable cups to accommodate changes in breast size.

8. Accessorize with Comfort in Mind: Accessorizing can elevate your pregnancy outfits while adding a personal touch. Opt for comfortable accessories like scarves,

statement jewelry, and stretchy belts that can enhance your look without compromising your comfort. Avoid accessories that may feel restrictive or tight around your belly.

Remember, the key to dressing stylishly and comfortably during pregnancy is to prioritize your comfort while expressing your unique sense of style. Embrace your changing body, experiment with different silhouettes and colors, and invest in clothing that makes you feel confident and beautiful. By curating a well-thought-out maternity wardrobe, you can navigate your pregnancy journey with style, comfort, and grace.

Chapter 8: Navigating the Medical Maze

As an expectant mother, navigating the medical system during pregnancy can be a daunting task. From choosing a healthcare provider to understanding medical procedures and interventions, it can be overwhelming to navigate this complex maze. However, it's essential to become informed about your options and feel confident in advocating for yourself and your baby's needs.

Understanding Prenatal Tests and Screenings

Understanding Prenatal Tests and Screenings

Prenatal tests and screenings play a vital role in monitoring the health and development of both you and your baby throughout pregnancy. These tests provide valuable information that can help identify any potential risks or conditions, allowing for early intervention and appropriate medical care. Understanding the purpose, benefits, and limitations of these tests empowers you to make informed decisions regarding your prenatal care. Let's delve into the details of prenatal tests and screenings to gain a comprehensive understanding.

1. Blood Tests:
Blood tests are a routine part of prenatal care and can provide essential information about your overall health and identify any underlying medical conditions that may impact your pregnancy. These tests typically include:

- Blood Type and Rh Factor: Determining your blood type and Rh factor is important to identify any potential blood incompatibilities between you and your baby.

- Complete Blood Count (CBC): This test measures different components of your blood, such as red blood cells, white blood cells, and platelets, to assess for conditions like anemia or infections.

- Blood Glucose Screening: This test helps identify gestational diabetes, a condition that affects blood sugar levels during pregnancy.

2. Genetic Screening:
Genetic screening tests assess the risk of specific genetic disorders or chromosomal abnormalities in your baby. These tests are optional and may include:

- Carrier Screening: This test determines if you and your partner carry genes for certain genetic conditions, such as cystic fibrosis or sickle cell anemia. It helps assess the likelihood of passing these conditions to your baby.

- Non-Invasive Prenatal Testing (NIPT): NIPT involves analyzing a sample of your blood to screen for common chromosomal abnormalities, such as Down syndrome, trisomy 18, and trisomy 13. This test has a high accuracy rate and can be performed as early as 10 weeks into pregnancy.

- Maternal Serum Screening (Quad Screen): This blood test is typically performed between 15 and 20 weeks of pregnancy and screens for the risk of chromosomal abnormalities and certain birth defects. It measures levels of various hormones and proteins in the mother's blood.

3. Ultrasound:
Ultrasound imaging uses sound waves to create pictures of your baby and the reproductive organs. Ultrasounds serve multiple purposes throughout pregnancy, including:

- Dating Ultrasound: This early ultrasound, typically performed in the first trimester, helps determine your baby's gestational age and estimate the due date.

- Nuchal Translucency Ultrasound: Usually performed between 11 and 14 weeks, this test assesses the thickness of the fluid at the back of the baby's neck. It helps identify the risk of chromosomal abnormalities, particularly Down syndrome.

- Anatomy Ultrasound: Conducted around 18-20 weeks, this detailed ultrasound examines the baby's anatomy, checking for any structural abnormalities or signs of potential complications.

4. Additional Screening and Diagnostic Tests:
Depending on your specific circumstances or identified risks, additional screening or diagnostic tests may be recommended, such as:

- Amniocentesis: This diagnostic test involves collecting a small amount of amniotic fluid for analysis. It can detect chromosomal abnormalities and genetic disorders with high accuracy but is usually offered to women at higher risk.

- Chorionic Villus Sampling (CVS): Similar to amniocentesis, CVS is a diagnostic test that involves obtaining a small sample of the placental tissue. It can detect genetic conditions and chromosomal abnormalities, and it's typically performed between 10 and 12 weeks of pregnancy.

- Fetal Doppler Monitoring: This non-invasive test uses a handheld device to listen to your baby's heartbeat. It helps assess the baby's well-being and monitor their heart rate and rhythm.

5. Group B Streptococcus (GBS) Testing:

Around the 36th week of pregnancy, you will be tested for Group B Streptococcus, a type of bacteria that can be present in the vagina or rectum. GBS testing is important as it helps determine if you are a carrier of this bacteria, which could be passed to your baby during childbirth. If positive, antibiotics can be administered during labor to prevent the baby from acquiring the infection.

6. Non-Stress Test (NST) and Biophysical Profile (BPP):

These tests are typically performed in the later stages of pregnancy to monitor your baby's well-being. The NST measures the baby's heart rate in response to their movements, while the BPP combines an ultrasound assessment with the NST to evaluate the baby's movements, breathing, muscle tone, amniotic fluid level, and heart rate patterns.

It's essential to discuss the purpose, benefits, and potential risks of each test with your healthcare provider. They will guide you in deciding which tests are appropriate for your specific situation and address any concerns or questions you may have. Remember, prenatal tests and screenings are designed to provide valuable information about your baby's health and well-being, giving you the opportunity to make informed decisions and seek appropriate care if necessary.

While these tests are essential, it's important to note that they have limitations and cannot guarantee the absence of all potential health issues. They are tools to aid in assessment and early detection, but not definitive diagnoses. If any abnormal results or concerns arise, further diagnostic testing or consultation with a specialist may be recommended.

By understanding the purpose and process of prenatal tests and screenings, you can actively participate in your prenatal care journey. Engage in open and honest discussions with your healthcare provider, ask questions, and voice any concerns you may have. Remember that the ultimate goal of these tests is to support the health and well-being of both you and your baby, ensuring a safe and positive pregnancy experience.

Making Informed Decisions about Medical Interventions

During pregnancy, you may encounter various medical interventions that aim to ensure the health and well-being of both you and your baby. These interventions can range from routine procedures to interventions that address specific concerns or complications. It's important to approach these decisions with an informed mindset, weighing the potential benefits, risks, and alternatives. By actively participating in the decision-making process, you can make choices that align with your preferences and values. Let's delve into the details of making informed decisions about medical interventions.

1. Gather Information:
Start by gathering information about the intervention being proposed. Consult reputable sources such as medical professionals, evidence-based literature, and trustworthy websites. Gain a clear understanding of the procedure, its purpose, potential benefits, risks, and alternatives.

2. Ask Questions:
During discussions with your healthcare provider, ask questions to clarify any uncertainties or concerns. Consider asking:

   - What is the specific intervention being recommended and why?
   - What are the potential benefits and risks associated with the intervention?
      - Are there any alternatives or non-invasive options to consider?

- What is the evidence supporting the use of this intervention?

- How does the intervention align with my birth preferences and values?

- Are there any potential long-term implications or effects on me or my baby?

- What happens if the intervention is declined or postponed?

3. Seek Second Opinions:
If you have reservations or doubts about a recommended intervention, don't hesitate to seek a second opinion. Consulting another healthcare provider can provide you with a different perspective and help you make a more informed decision.

4. Consider Personal Circumstances:
Evaluate your personal circumstances and medical history when making decisions about interventions. Each pregnancy is unique, and factors such as your health, previous experiences, and current condition may influence the appropriateness of certain

interventions. Take into account your specific situation and consult with your healthcare provider regarding the potential benefits and risks in your case.

5. Assess the Evidence:
Examine the available evidence related to the intervention in question. Look for research studies, clinical guidelines, and recommendations from reputable medical organizations. Evaluate the quality of the evidence and consider whether it aligns with your preferences and values. It's important to remember that evidence can vary, and what may be suitable for one person may not be the best choice for another.

6. Discuss with Your Birth Partner or Support Person:
Engage in open and honest discussions with your birth partner or support person. Share the information you have gathered, discuss your concerns, and consider their input. Having a trusted person by your side

can provide valuable insights and support in the decision-making process.

7. Trust Your Instincts:
Ultimately, trust your instincts and intuition. You know yourself and your body best. Consider your gut feelings and listen to what resonates with you. If something doesn't feel right or align with your values, it's important to communicate your concerns and explore alternative options.

8. Maintain Open Communication:
Maintaining open communication with your healthcare provider is crucial throughout the decision-making process. Express your thoughts, concerns, and preferences clearly. A collaborative approach allows you to work together in making decisions that prioritize both your and your baby's well-being.

Remember that making informed decisions about medical interventions is a personal and individual process. What works for one person may not work for another. Trust yourself and your ability to make choices that feel right for you and your baby. By actively participating in the decision-making process and seeking information, you can navigate the realm of medical interventions with confidence and ensure that your pregnancy journey aligns with your preferences and values.

Advocating for Your Birth Plan and Preferences

Your birth plan represents your desires and preferences for how you envision your childbirth experience. It serves as a valuable tool to communicate your wishes to your healthcare providers and support team. Advocating for your birth plan and preferences empowers you to actively participate in decision-making, maintain control over your birth experience, and promote a positive and empowering journey. Let's explore effective strategies for advocating for your birth plan and preferences.

1. Educate Yourself:

Start by educating yourself about the birthing process, available options, and interventions. Attend childbirth classes, read books, and gather information from reputable sources. The more knowledge you have, the better equipped you'll be to advocate for your preferences and make informed decisions.

2. Communicate Early and Clearly:

Initiate conversations about your birth plan and preferences early in your prenatal care. Discuss your desires with your healthcare provider and ensure they understand your goals. Clearly articulate what is important to you, whether it's a specific birthing position, pain management techniques, or preferences for immediate skin-to-skin contact. Provide a written copy of your birth plan and review it with your healthcare provider.

3. Build a Supportive Birth Team:
Surround yourself with a supportive birth team who understands and respects your wishes. Your birth partner, doula, or other support persons should be familiar with your birth plan and prepared to advocate for your preferences during labor. Their presence can provide emotional support and help ensure your voice is heard.

4. Establish Trusting Relationships:
Develop trusting relationships with your healthcare providers. Open and respectful communication is essential in fostering a collaborative environment where your preferences are valued. Seek healthcare providers who align with your birth philosophy and have a track record of supporting personalized birth plans.

5. Discuss Your Birth Plan with the Hospital
or Birth Center:
If you plan to give birth in a hospital or birth
center, schedule a meeting or tour to
discuss your birth plan with the staff. Inquire
about their policies and practices, and
ensure they are supportive of your
preferences. Address any concerns or
potential conflicts in advance.

6. Understand Your Rights and Options:
Familiarize yourself with your rights as a
birthing person. Know that you have the
right to make informed decisions and have
those decisions respected. Be aware of the
various options available to you during labor
and birth, including pain management
techniques, movement restrictions, and
monitoring preferences. Understanding your
rights empowers you to advocate for your
choices confidently.

7. Practice Effective Communication:

During labor, clearly communicate your preferences to your healthcare team. Assertively express your desires, concerns, and any changes to your birth plan. Use "I" statements to express your needs, such as "I would like to try different positions for pushing" or "I prefer to delay cord clamping."

8. Utilize Supportive Techniques:
Enlist the support of your birth partner or doula to help advocate for your birth plan. They can remind healthcare providers of your preferences, offer suggestions, and provide emotional support. Additionally, practicing relaxation techniques, breathing exercises, and visualization can help you stay focused and calm, enhancing your ability to advocate for your preferences effectively.

9. Be Flexible and Open-minded:
While it's important to advocate for your birth plan, it's also crucial to remain

open-minded and flexible. Birth can be unpredictable, and unexpected circumstances may arise. In such cases, understanding the medical rationale behind recommendations and being open to alternative approaches can help you make informed decisions that prioritize the health and safety of you and your baby.

10. Reflect on Your Birth Experience:
After your birth, take time to reflect on your experience and evaluate how well your birth plan was followed. Share feedback with your healthcare providers and consider discussing your experience with other expectant parents or support groups. Reflecting on your experience can help you refine your birth plan for future pregnancies and empower you to advocate even more effectively.

11. Seek Professional Support:
If you encounter challenges or feel that your birth plan was not adequately respected,

consider seeking support from a professional advocate or a birth rights organization. They can provide guidance, resources, and help navigate any potential concerns or conflicts.

12. Share Your Experience:
Sharing your birth story with others can be a powerful way to raise awareness and inspire other expectant parents. Your experience can shed light on the importance of advocating for birth plans and encourage others to do the same. Whether through personal conversations, online platforms, or participating in support groups, your story can make a difference.

Remember, advocating for your birth plan and preferences is about taking an active role in shaping your birth experience. It is your right to be an active participant, making informed decisions that align with your values and desires. By educating yourself, establishing trusting relationships, and effectively communicating your preferences, you can assert your voice and create an environment that supports your birth vision. Through careful planning, open dialogue, and a supportive birth team, you can navigate the birthing process with confidence, knowing that your choices are respected and honored.

Chapter 9: Preparing for Labor and Delivery

Bringing new life into the world is a remarkable and transformative experience, and preparing for labor and delivery is an essential part of the journey toward meeting your precious baby. As an expectant parent, it is natural to feel a mix of excitement, anticipation, and perhaps a touch of apprehension. But fear not, for this chapter is dedicated to equipping you with the knowledge, tools, and resources you need to navigate the path of labor and delivery with confidence and ease.

Preparing for labor and delivery goes beyond just the physical aspects of childbirth. It involves embracing the emotional, mental, and spiritual aspects of this transformative process. It is about understanding the changes your body will undergo, learning about the various stages of labor, exploring pain management techniques, making informed decisions, and creating a birth plan that aligns with your wishes and desires. It is also about cultivating a mindset of trust, strength, and resilience as you embark on this awe-inspiring journey.

Educating Yourself about Different Birthing Options

One of the most empowering steps you can take in preparing for labor and delivery is to educate yourself about the different birthing options available to you. Each individual has unique preferences, values, and circumstances that may influence the ideal approach to childbirth. By familiarizing yourself with various birthing options, you can make informed decisions that align with your desires and promote a positive birth experience. Let's delve into the details of different birthing options and how you can educate yourself about them.

1. Hospital Birth:

Hospital births are the most common and traditional option for childbirth. Hospitals offer a range of medical interventions, including pain management options and access to specialized care in case of complications. Educate yourself about the policies, practices, and available amenities at the hospitals in your area. Attend hospital tours, prenatal classes, and childbirth education programs offered by the hospital to gain a better understanding of the environment and protocols.

2. Birth Center:

Birth centers provide a homelike setting for labor and delivery, often with a focus on natural childbirth. They offer a middle ground between home birth and hospital birth, providing a supportive and non-medicalized environment. Research local birth centers, inquire about their philosophies, and consider attending open houses or consultations to get a feel for their approach to childbirth. Understand the services they provide, such as water births, midwifery care, and postpartum support.

3. Home Birth:

Home birth involves giving birth in the comfort of your own home, supported by a certified professional midwife or a qualified healthcare provider. It offers a familiar and intimate setting where you can create a personalized birth experience. If you are considering a home birth, seek out licensed home birth midwives, understand their qualifications, and discuss their protocols and emergency plans. Research the safety statistics and outcomes associated with home birth in your region to make an informed decision.

4. Midwifery Care:

Midwives are healthcare professionals who specialize in supporting women during pregnancy, labor, and birth. They provide personalized care, emphasizing a holistic and woman-centered approach. Educate yourself about the different types of midwives, such as certified nurse-midwives (CNMs), certified professional midwives (CPMs), and direct-entry midwives. Research their scope of practice, qualifications, and the settings in which they practice, whether it be hospitals, birth centers, or home births.

5. Water Birth:
Water birth involves laboring and giving birth in a birthing pool or tub filled with warm water. This option provides a soothing and buoyant environment that may help ease pain and promote relaxation. Learn about the benefits and considerations of water birth, including the availability of water birthing facilities, safety measures, and how

to find healthcare providers experienced in supporting water births.

6. Doula Support:
Doulas are trained professionals who provide emotional, physical, and informational support to birthing individuals and their partners. They offer continuous support throughout labor and delivery, advocating for your preferences and helping you navigate the birthing process. Research the benefits of doula support, explore different types of doulas (such as birth doulas, postpartum doulas, and sibling doulas), and consider attending doula informational sessions or workshops.

7. Alternative Birthing Techniques:
Beyond conventional options, there are alternative birthing techniques that you may find intriguing, such as hypnobirthing, acupuncture, acupressure, aromatherapy, and chiropractic care. Educate yourself about these techniques, their potential

benefits, and how they can be integrated into your birth plan. Consult with qualified practitioners in these fields to discuss their approach to supporting childbirth.

To educate yourself about these different birthing options, consider the following steps:

- Read books, articles, and reputable online resources that provide information about various birthing options. Look for evidence-based materials that present a balanced view and include personal stories and experiences.
- Attend prenatal classes and workshops that cover different birthing options. These classes are often led by childbirth educators, doulas, or midwives who can provide valuable insights and answer your questions.
- Seek recommendations and referrals from trusted healthcare professionals, friends, or family members who have had positive

experiences with specific birthing options. Hearing firsthand accounts can help you gather more information and perspectives.

- Join online forums, social media groups, or local support groups focused on pregnancy and childbirth. Engage in conversations with other expectant parents who have explored different birthing options. Learn from their experiences and ask questions to gain a broader understanding.

- Arrange consultations or interviews with healthcare providers who specialize in the birthing options you are considering. This will allow you to discuss your preferences, ask specific questions, and assess their compatibility with your desired birth experience.

- Consider hiring a birth doula who can provide guidance and support in exploring different birthing options. Doulas often have extensive knowledge and experience working with diverse birthing preferences and can help you navigate the decision-making process.

Remember, the purpose of educating yourself about different birthing options is not to overwhelm yourself with information or feel pressured to choose a particular path. Rather, it is about understanding the range of possibilities available to you, considering your own preferences and values, and making choices that resonate with your unique circumstances. By becoming well-informed, you can approach your birth experience with confidence, knowing that you have explored the options and made decisions that align with your desires for a positive and empowering journey into parenthood.

Creating a Birth Plan that Aligns with Your Desires

A birth plan is a powerful tool that allows you to communicate your preferences and desires for your labor, delivery, and postpartum experience. It helps you assert your voice, ensure that your wishes are respected, and promote a positive and personalized birth journey. Creating a birth plan involves thoughtful consideration, open communication with your healthcare provider, and a clear understanding of your options. Let's explore the steps involved in creating a birth plan that aligns with your desires.

1. Research and Reflect:
Begin by researching the various aspects of labor and delivery. Educate yourself about pain management options, medical interventions, labor positions, postpartum care, and any specific practices or policies of the birthing facility or healthcare provider you have chosen. Reflect on your values, preferences, and goals for your birth experience. Consider what matters most to you and what type of atmosphere, support, and interventions you are comfortable with.

2. Communicate with your Healthcare Provider:
Open and ongoing communication with your healthcare provider is crucial in creating a birth plan that aligns with your desires. Schedule a prenatal appointment specifically to discuss your birth preferences. Share your research, ask questions, and express your concerns and hopes. Collaborate with your healthcare provider to ensure that your birth plan is realistic and feasible given your medical history, any potential complications, and the policies of the birthing facility.

3. Choose Your Support Team:
Think about who you want to have by your side during labor and delivery. This could include your partner, family members, friends, or a doula. Discuss their roles and responsibilities, as well as their involvement in decision-making processes. Your support team should be aware of your birth plan and

be prepared to advocate for your preferences during labor.

4. Outline Your Preferences:
Write down your birth plan in a clear and concise manner. Begin with a brief introduction that highlights your overarching goals and values for the birth experience. Then, outline your preferences for various aspects, such as pain management, labor positions, monitoring, fetal interventions, and postpartum care. Consider including information about your desired atmosphere, music or aromatherapy preferences, and any cultural or religious practices you would like to incorporate.

5. Flexibility and Alternative Options:
While it is important to have a birth plan, it is equally crucial to remain flexible and open to alternative options. Labor and delivery can be unpredictable, and unexpected circumstances may arise that require deviation from the original plan. Include a

section in your birth plan that acknowledges this and expresses your willingness to consider alternative options as long as they are discussed and explained to you in advance.

6. Discuss and Review:
Schedule a follow-up appointment with your healthcare provider to discuss and review your birth plan. Ensure that all parties involved are clear on the contents of the plan and that any questions or concerns are addressed. This is also an opportunity to make adjustments or revisions based on new information or discussions.

7. Share Your Birth Plan:
Provide copies of your birth plan to your healthcare provider, your support team, and the birthing facility where you plan to deliver. Make sure that your preferences are known and that your birth plan is included in your medical records. Discuss your birth plan with the nursing staff upon arrival at the

birthing facility so that they are aware of your preferences.

8. Prepare for Unexpected Situations:
Although you may have a clear birth plan, it is essential to mentally and emotionally prepare for unexpected situations or changes in circumstances. Educate yourself about alternative options and interventions that may arise. This will help you maintain a sense of calm and adaptability during the labor process.

Remember, a birth plan is a flexible guide, not a rigid set of demands. It serves as a way to express your desires and preferences, promote open communication with your healthcare team,and ensure that your wishes are considered during the birth process. Here are a few additional considerations to keep in mind as you create your birth plan:

9. Be Specific and Clear:

When outlining your preferences, be as specific and clear as possible. Use simple language and avoid medical jargon. Include details such as preferred positions for labor and pushing, whether you want to use a birthing ball or water immersion for pain management, and any specific comfort measures you would like to incorporate, such as massage or relaxation techniques. This clarity will help your healthcare team understand your desires more effectively.

10. Prioritize Your Preferences:
Identify the aspects of your birth experience that are most important to you. Prioritize these preferences and highlight them in your birth plan. For example, if having immediate skin-to-skin contact with your baby after birth is crucial to you, emphasize this in your plan. By highlighting your top priorities, you ensure that they receive particular attention and consideration.

11. Consider Contingency Plans:

While you may have a specific vision for your birth experience, it is essential to consider alternative plans in case circumstances deviate from your initial expectations. Discuss backup options with your healthcare provider and include them in your birth plan. This might involve interventions such as induction, assisted delivery, or cesarean section. By acknowledging these possibilities and discussing them in advance, you can maintain a sense of control and preparedness.

12. Review and Revise Regularly:
As your pregnancy progresses, take the time to review and revise your birth plan if necessary. Preferences may change as you gather more information, receive new medical advice, or simply evolve in your understanding of your own desires. Keep an open line of communication with your healthcare provider and discuss any

changes or adjustments to your birth plan during your prenatal appointments.

13. Be Open to Dialogue:
Approach your birth plan as a starting point for dialogue and collaboration with your healthcare team. While you have the right to express your desires, remember that your healthcare provider has the expertise to ensure the safety and well-being of you and your baby. Remain open to their recommendations and explanations, and engage in meaningful discussions about the best course of action.

14. Advocate for Yourself:
During labor and delivery, stay actively involved in the decision-making process. Your birth plan serves as a tool to help you communicate your preferences, but it is up to you to assert your needs and desires during the birthing process. If any deviations from your plan are proposed, ask questions,

seek clarification, and discuss potential alternatives.

Creating a birth plan that aligns with your desires empowers you to actively participate in your birth experience. It encourages open communication with your healthcare team and ensures that your voice is heard and respected. Remember, birth plans are not set in stone, and flexibility is key. Trust in your ability to make informed decisions and embrace the journey of childbirth with confidence and positivity.

Practicing Relaxation Techniques and Pain Management Strategies

During labor and delivery, it is normal to experience various levels of discomfort and pain. However, there are effective relaxation techniques and pain management strategies that can help you cope with these sensations and create a more positive birthing experience. By incorporating these techniques into your birth preparation, you can enhance your ability to relax, manage pain, and remain calm throughout the process. Let's explore some of these techniques in detail:

1. Deep Breathing:
Deep breathing is a fundamental relaxation technique that helps you focus your attention, regulate your breathing patterns, and promote a sense of calm. Practice deep breathing exercises during pregnancy to become familiar with the technique. During labor, use slow, deep breaths to stay centered and relaxed, particularly during contractions. Take long, slow breaths in through your nose, filling your abdomen with air, and exhale slowly through your mouth. Deep breathing can help alleviate tension and reduce anxiety.

2. Visualization and Guided Imagery:
Visualization and guided imagery techniques involve creating mental images

that promote relaxation and focus. Close your eyes and imagine yourself in a peaceful, serene environment, such as a beach or a garden. Visualize the sensations of relaxation, envisioning each muscle in your body releasing tension. You can also use guided imagery recordings or apps specifically designed for childbirth to help guide your visualization process.

3. Progressive Muscle Relaxation:
Progressive muscle relaxation involves systematically tensing and releasing different muscle groups in your body to achieve deep relaxation. Start from your toes and work your way up to your head, progressively tensing and then releasing each muscle group. This technique promotes physical and mental relaxation and can be particularly helpful during the early stages of labor.

4. Positioning and Movement:

Experiment with different labor positions and movements to find what feels most comfortable for you. Changing positions frequently during labor can help relieve pain and encourage optimal fetal positioning. Some common positions include standing, walking, squatting, sitting on a birthing ball, or using a support bar for leverage. Listen to your body and trust your instincts in finding positions that alleviate discomfort.

5. Water Immersion:

Water immersion, such as taking a warm bath or shower, can provide significant pain relief during labor. The buoyancy of the water helps alleviate the pressure on your joints and promotes relaxation. Many birthing facilities offer birthing tubs or showers specifically designed for laboring women. Discuss the option of water immersion with your healthcare provider and include it in your birth plan if it aligns with your preferences.

6. Massage and Counterpressure:
Massage can be a powerful tool for pain relief during labor. Gentle massage applied to your lower back, hips, or shoulders by your partner or a doula can help release tension and promote relaxation. Additionally, applying counterpressure to your lower back during contractions can help alleviate pain. Experiment with different massage techniques and pressure points to find what works best for you.

7. Distraction and Visualization Tools:
Utilize distraction techniques and visualization tools to redirect your focus during labor. This could include listening to soothing music, using aromatherapy with essential oils, or watching calming visuals on a screen or projection. These tools can help shift your attention away from pain sensations and create a more relaxed and positive atmosphere.

8. Acupressure and Acupuncture:

Acupressure and acupuncture involve applying gentle pressure or using thin needles on specific points of the body to alleviate pain and promote relaxation. Some women find these techniques helpful for managing labor pain. If you are interested in using acupressure or acupuncture, consult with a certified practitioner who specializes in prenatal care.

9. Medication and Medical Interventions:
In some cases, medication or medical interventions may be necessary for pain management during labor. These options can include epidurals, nitrous oxide, or intravenous pain medications. It is important to discuss these options with your healthcare provider beforehand, so you are informed about the benefits, risks, and potential side effects. If you prefer a medication-free birth, communicate your desires clearly in your birth plan and discuss alternative pain management strategies with your healthcare provider.

10. Continuous Support:
Having continuous support during labor, such as a partner, family member, or doula, can significantly contribute to your comfort and emotional well-being. They can provide physical and emotional support, remind you of relaxation techniques, and advocate for your needs. Their presence can help you feel more secure and confident in managing pain.

Remember, every woman's experience of labor and pain is unique, and what works for one person may not work for another. It is essential to explore and practice different relaxation techniques and pain management strategies during your pregnancy to determine which ones resonate with you. Attend childbirth education classes, seek guidance from your healthcare provider, and connect with experienced mothers to learn about their coping strategies.

Preparing yourself mentally and physically for labor and delivery is an empowering process that can positively influence your birth experience. By practicing relaxation techniques and pain management strategies, you can navigate the intensity of labor with greater ease, maintain a sense of control, and enhance your overall well-being. Trust in your body's ability to birth your baby and surround yourself with a supportive birth team that honors and respects your choices.

As you embark on this chapter of your pregnancy, remember that each birth experience is unique, and there is no one-size-fits-all approach. This section will provide you with the information and tools you need to make informed choices, adapt to unexpected circumstances, and embark on this extraordinary journey with confidence and grace. Embrace the transformative power of labor and delivery, knowing that you are well-prepared to welcome your little one into the world.

Chapter 10: Postpartum Preparation

While pregnancy and childbirth are often the focus of attention during the journey to motherhood, it is equally important to prepare for the transformative and beautiful phase that follows: the postpartum period. The postpartum period, often referred to as the fourth trimester, is a time of adjustment, healing, and bonding with your newborn. It is a time when you need ample support, self-care, and practical preparations to navigate this new chapter with confidence and grace.

From physical recovery to emotional adjustments and the demands of caring for a newborn, the postpartum period is a multifaceted experience that requires thoughtful planning and support. It is a time when you need to prioritize self-care, seek assistance from loved ones, and build a network of support that can help you navigate the challenges and joys of early motherhood.

Anticipating the Physical and Emotional Changes After Birth

The postpartum period is a time of significant physical and emotional changes as your body adjusts to the demands of childbirth and you navigate the joys and challenges of motherhood. Understanding and anticipating these changes can help you prepare mentally and emotionally, allowing you to approach this transformative time with a sense of empowerment and resilience. Let's explore in detail the physical and emotional changes you may experience after giving birth:

1. Physical Changes:

a. Postpartum Bleeding: After giving birth, you will experience vaginal bleeding known as lochia. This bleeding is similar to a heavy menstrual period and can last for several weeks. Initially, the bleeding may be bright red and gradually transition to a lighter color. It's important to use sanitary pads rather than tampons during this time to avoid the risk of infection.

b. Uterine Contractions: Your uterus will undergo contractions known as afterpains as it returns to its pre-pregnancy size. These contractions can be more pronounced during breastfeeding, as breastfeeding triggers the release of the hormone oxytocin, which stimulates uterine contractions. Over-the-counter pain relievers, warm compresses, or relaxation techniques can help alleviate discomfort.

c. Breast Changes: Your breasts will undergo significant changes as they prepare for breastfeeding. Initially, your breasts may feel tender, swollen, and engorged. As your milk production regulates, you may experience leaking, fluctuating breast size, and nipple soreness. Wearing a supportive bra, using warm or cold compresses, and seeking guidance from a lactation consultant can help manage these changes.

d. Vaginal Changes: If you had a vaginal birth, you may experience soreness, swelling, and possible tears or episiotomy incisions. It is essential to keep the perineal area clean and practice good hygiene to promote healing. Using warm sitz baths, applying ice packs, and using pain-relieving sprays or creams can help alleviate discomfort. If you had a cesarean birth, you will have an incision that requires proper care and monitoring for signs of infection.

e. Hormonal Shifts: Hormonal fluctuations after birth can contribute to emotional changes and physical symptoms. Estrogen and progesterone levels drop significantly, which can lead to mood swings, fatigue, and even postpartum blues or depression. It's important to reach out to your healthcare provider if you experience persistent feelings of sadness, anxiety, or depression.

2. Emotional Changes:

a. Baby Blues: It is common for many women to experience the baby blues within the first few days after giving birth. You may feel teary, emotional, and overwhelmed. These feelings are typically transient and resolve within a couple of weeks. Engaging in self-care, seeking support from loved ones, and connecting with other new mothers can help you navigate this emotional transition.

b. Postpartum Depression: Some women may experience postpartum depression, which is a more severe and prolonged form of mood disturbance. Symptoms may include persistent feelings of sadness, loss of interest or pleasure in activities, changes in appetite, sleep disturbances, and difficulty bonding with the baby. It is important to seek professional help if you suspect you may be experiencing postpartum depression.

c. Fatigue and Sleep Changes: Sleep deprivation is common during the early weeks and months of motherhood. Frequent nighttime feedings and adjusting to a newborn's sleep patterns can leave you feeling exhausted. Prioritizing rest, taking naps when possible, and accepting help from others can help manage fatigue and promote overall well-being.

d. Body Image and Self-esteem: Your body undergoes remarkable changes during pregnancy and childbirth. Adjusting to your postpartum body can be challenging, and you may have concerns about weight and stretch marks.

After giving birth, it's normal to experience physical and emotional changes. Understanding and anticipating these changes can help you prepare and cope during the postpartum period.

It's essential to remember that these changes are normal and temporary, and seeking support from your partner, family, friends, or healthcare professionals can help you navigate this period.

Preparing for postpartum recovery also involves planning for practical matters such as arranging for help with household chores, meals, and childcare. Taking care of yourself during this time is crucial to your overall recovery and well-being. It's essential to get adequate rest, eat a healthy diet, and stay hydrated.

In the next sections of this book, we will discuss ways to take care of yourself during the postpartum period and strategies to manage physical and emotional changes.

Remember that reaching out for support and asking for help when needed is a sign of strength, not weakness.

Planning for Postpartum Recovery and Self-Care

The postpartum period is a time of immense change and adjustment, both physically and emotionally. Planning for your postpartum recovery and prioritizing self-care is crucial to support your healing, well-being, and the bonding experience with your baby. Here are some key aspects to consider when planning for postpartum recovery and self-care:

1. Rest and Sleep:
Rest and sleep are essential for your physical and mental recovery after childbirth. However, with the demands of a newborn, it can be challenging to get uninterrupted sleep. Plan ahead by creating a comfortable sleep environment,

establishing a nighttime routine, and discussing sleep arrangements with your partner or support person. Take advantage of daytime naps whenever possible and delegate household chores to others to allow yourself adequate rest.

2. Nutrition and Hydration:
Proper nutrition is vital for your postpartum recovery, especially if you are breastfeeding. Plan for nourishing meals and snacks that are easy to prepare and rich in nutrients. Stock up on healthy, pre-prepared options or consider meal delivery services. Stay hydrated by drinking plenty of water throughout the day, as breastfeeding and recovery can be dehydrating.

3. Pain Management:
During postpartum recovery, it's common to experience discomfort, such as perineal soreness, breast engorgement, or uterine cramping. Discuss pain management

options with your healthcare provider and have necessary supplies, such as pain relievers, soothing creams, and ice packs, readily available. Utilize relaxation techniques, warm baths, and gentle stretching to alleviate discomfort.

4. Perineal Care:

If you had a vaginal birth, taking care of your perineal area is crucial for healing. Practice good hygiene by using warm water for cleansing after using the bathroom and patting the area dry. Consider using a peri bottle to gently cleanse the area after urination. Applying witch hazel pads or using sitz baths can provide soothing relief. Wearing loose-fitting, breathable underwear and using sanitary pads designed for postpartum use can enhance comfort.

5. Breast Care:

If you choose to breastfeed, establishing a good breastfeeding routine and taking care of your breasts is essential. Learn proper latching techniques and seek guidance from a lactation consultant if needed. Ensure proper breast support with well-fitting nursing bras or tops. If you experience nipple soreness or engorgement, applying warm or cold compresses, using lanolin cream, or expressing a small amount of milk can offer relief.

6. Emotional Support:
The postpartum period can be emotionally challenging as you adjust to your new role as a mother. Reach out to your partner, family, or friends for emotional support and understanding. Joining support groups or online communities with other new mothers can provide valuable connections and reassurance. If you're experiencing intense or prolonged feelings of sadness, anxiety, or mood changes, don't hesitate to seek professional help.

7. Bonding with Your Baby:

Creating a nurturing and loving bond with your newborn is an essential part of postpartum recovery. Spend quality time with your baby, engage in skin-to-skin contact, and practice gentle touch and soothing techniques. Take advantage of quiet moments to connect through eye contact, talking, and singing to your baby. Bonding promotes emotional well-being for both you and your little one.

8. Self-Care Rituals:
Carve out time for self-care activities that bring you joy and relaxation. It can be as simple as taking a warm bath, reading a book, listening to music, practicing deep breathing or mindfulness exercises, or engaging in a hobby you love. Consider enlisting the help of your partner, family, or friends to allow yourself regular moments of self-care.

9. Ask for Help:

Remember that it's okay to ask for help and delegate tasks during the postpartum period. Don't hesitate to reach out to your support network when you need assistance with household chores, meal preparation, or caring for your baby. Communicate your needs clearly and accept help graciously. Surrounding yourself with a supportive community can make a significant difference in your postpartum recovery and overall well-being.

10. Adjusting Expectations:
Be gentle with yourself and remember that the postpartum period is a time of adjustment and learning. It's normal to feel overwhelmed or unsure at times. Allow yourself to adapt to your new role as a mother at your own pace. Don't compare your journey to others and embrace the unique experience that is unfolding for you and your baby.

11. Communicate with Your Healthcare Provider:

Stay in regular contact with your healthcare provider during the postpartum period. Attend scheduled check-ups to monitor your recovery, address any concerns, and receive guidance on postpartum care. Don't hesitate to reach out if you have questions or if something doesn't feel right. Your healthcare provider is there to support you on your postpartum journey.

Remember, postpartum recovery is a process that takes time. Be patient and kind to yourself as you navigate the physical and emotional changes that come with motherhood. By planning ahead, prioritizing self-care, and seeking support, you can lay the foundation for a positive and fulfilling postpartum experience. Embrace this transformative time, allowing yourself to heal, bond with your baby, and embark on the beautiful journey of motherhood.

Building a Support System for the Postpartum Period

The postpartum period can be both exhilarating and challenging as you navigate the physical and emotional changes that come with new motherhood. Having a strong support system in place can make a significant difference in your well-being and adjustment during this time. Here are some key strategies for building a support system for the postpartum period:

1. Partner or Spouse:
Your partner or spouse plays a crucial role in providing support during the postpartum period. Open and honest communication is essential in discussing your needs, fears, and expectations. Encourage your partner to participate in baby care activities, such as diaper changes and soothing the baby. Working together as a team can help alleviate the workload and provide emotional support for both of you.

2. Family and Close Friends:
Reach out to your immediate family members and close friends to let them know about your needs and ask for their support. They can assist with household chores, meal preparation, or taking care of older children if applicable. Having loved ones available to lend a helping hand can give you valuable time to rest, bond with your baby, or focus on self-care.

3. Postpartum Doula:
Consider hiring a postpartum doula who can provide practical and emotional support during the postpartum period. Postpartum doulas are trained professionals who offer assistance with newborn care, breastfeeding support, light household chores, and emotional guidance. They can provide valuable insights, reassurance, and expertise as you navigate the early days and weeks of motherhood.

4. Online Support Communities:
Joining online support communities or forums for new mothers can provide a sense of belonging and connection. These platforms allow you to share experiences, ask questions, and receive support from other women going through similar journeys. Online communities provide a safe space to discuss concerns, seek advice, and celebrate milestones, even during late-night feedings or moments of solitude.

5. Breastfeeding Support:
If you choose to breastfeed, seek out breastfeeding support groups, lactation consultants, or breastfeeding clinics in your community. These resources can provide valuable guidance, address concerns, and offer tips and techniques for successful breastfeeding. Connecting with other breastfeeding mothers can create a sense of camaraderie and shared experiences.

6. Postpartum Exercise Groups:

Participating in postpartum exercise groups or classes specifically designed for new mothers can offer numerous benefits. Not only does exercise contribute to physical well-being, but it also provides an opportunity to connect with other women who understand the challenges of postpartum recovery. These groups can foster a sense of camaraderie, motivation, and support as you work towards regaining strength and fitness.

7. Mental Health Professionals:
If you find yourself struggling with postpartum mood disorders, anxiety, or depression, seeking help from mental health professionals is essential. Connect with therapists or counselors experienced in perinatal mental health who can provide the support and guidance you need. Therapy sessions can offer a safe space to explore and process your emotions, develop coping strategies, and ensure your mental well-being.

8. Community Resources:

Explore community resources available for new mothers and families. Many areas offer parent-child playgroups, new parent support programs, breastfeeding cafes, or parenting classes. These resources provide opportunities to meet other parents, share experiences, and access educational support. Local libraries, hospitals, or community centers often host such programs.

Remember that building a support system takes time and effort. Start by identifying individuals or resources that align with your needs and values. Be open and willing to ask for help when you need it, as people around you often want to offer support but may not know how best to assist you. Surrounding yourself with a supportive network can provide encouragement, guidance, and a sense of community during the postpartum period.

By delving into these aspects of postpartum preparation, you will gain valuable insights and practical strategies to make the most of this transformative period. Remember, each postpartum journey is unique, and it's essential to trust your instincts and adopt these suggestions to fit your own needs and circumstances.

As you embark on the postpartum journey, embrace the beauty of this time, celebrate your strengths, and allow yourself to be supported and nurtured. By prioritizing self-care, seeking assistance when needed, and fostering a positive and loving environment, you will lay the groundwork for a joyful and fulfilling postpartum experience.

Chapter 11: Embracing Motherhood

Becoming a mother is a transformative and life-altering experience. It is a journey filled with love, joy, challenges, and personal growth. Embracing motherhood means embracing the profound changes that come with nurturing and raising a child. It is about discovering the depths of your strength, resilience, and capacity for unconditional love.

Motherhood is a unique journey for each woman, as every mother and child relationship is a beautiful individual. It is a journey that begins during pregnancy and continues throughout a lifetime. From the first flutter of life within the womb to the first steps, words, and milestones of your child, motherhood encompasses a range of emotions and experiences.

Embracing motherhood means embracing the privilege and responsibility of guiding a new life, shaping values, and fostering growth. It means celebrating the small victories, cherishing precious moments, and navigating the inevitable challenges with grace and resilience. Motherhood is a delicate balance of nurturing and letting go, of offering guidance while allowing your child to become their unique self.

Adapting to the Demands and Joys of Motherhood

Motherhood is a multifaceted role that demands flexibility, patience, and adaptability. It is a journey filled with both challenges and immense joys. Adapting to the demands of motherhood means navigating the ever-changing landscape of caring for a child while finding balance and fulfillment in your own life. Here are some key aspects to consider as you adapt to the demands and joys of motherhood:

1. Embracing the New Normal:
Motherhood brings about a new normal in your life. It involves adjusting to new routines, sleep patterns, and responsibilities. Embrace the changes and allow yourself time to adapt. Recognize that it is normal to feel overwhelmed or uncertain in the beginning. Be patient with yourself as you find your rhythm and establish a sense of normalcy within your new role as a mother.

2. Prioritizing Self-Care:
Self-care is vital as you adapt to the demands of motherhood. It is not selfish to take care of yourself; it is necessary for your well-being and ability to care for your child effectively. Prioritize activities that rejuvenate and recharge you, whether it's taking a hot bath, reading a book, practicing

mindfulness, or engaging in hobbies you enjoy. Remember that self-care looks different for everyone, so find what works best for you and make it a priority.

3. Establishing Boundaries:
Motherhood can come with numerous demands and expectations from others. It is important to establish clear boundaries to protect your time, energy, and mental well-being. Learn to say no when necessary and set realistic expectations for yourself. Communicate your needs and limits to your loved ones, and don't be afraid to ask for help when needed. Creating boundaries allows you to prioritize what truly matters and maintain a healthy balance in your life.

4. Seeking Support:
Building a support system is essential for adapting to the demands of motherhood. Surround yourself with people who understand and support you in your role as a mother. Seek out fellow moms, join

support groups, or connect with online communities where you can share experiences, seek advice, and gain support. Having a support network provides a sense of belonging, validation, and encouragement during challenging times.

5. Embracing Flexibility:
Motherhood requires flexibility as each day brings new surprises and challenges. Babies and children have their own unique schedules and needs that may differ from your expectations. Embrace the need for flexibility and adaptability in your daily routine. Being open to change and adjusting your plans as needed can help alleviate stress and create a more harmonious environment for both you and your child.

6. Embracing the Joys:
While motherhood comes with its share of demands, it is also a journey filled with incredible joys and rewards. Embrace and savor the precious moments with your child.

Take time to appreciate the small milestones, the giggles, the cuddles, and the love that fills your heart. Allow yourself to be present in the joyous moments and find gratitude in the journey of motherhood.

7. Embracing Imperfection:
Remember that no one is a perfect mother, and that's okay. Embrace the imperfections and embrace the learning process that comes with being a mom. Accept that there will be good days and challenging days, and that it's all part of the journey. Give yourself grace and compassion as you navigate the demands of motherhood, knowing that you are doing your best.

Adapting to the demands and joys of motherhood is a continuous process. It requires patience, self-reflection, and a willingness to learn and grow. Embrace the journey, be kind to yourself, and celebrate the beautiful moments that come with the privilege of being a mother. Remember, you are not alone on this path of motherhood. Reach out for support when you need it, lean on your loved ones, and connect with other mothers who can share their experiences and wisdom. Remember that every mother's journey is unique, and what works for one may not work for another. Trust your instincts and make decisions that align with your values and the needs of your family.

As you adapt to the demands of motherhood, be mindful of the importance of self-care. Take time to nourish your own physical, emotional, and mental well-being. Prioritize activities that bring you joy and rejuvenation. Whether it's taking a walk in nature, practicing yoga, reading a book, or engaging in a creative outlet, carving out time for yourself is crucial in maintaining balance and replenishing your energy.

Additionally, embrace the power of self-compassion. Motherhood can be challenging, and it's normal to experience moments of doubt, guilt, or exhaustion. Be gentle with yourself and practice self-compassion when facing difficulties. Remember that you are doing the best you can with the resources and knowledge you have. Give yourself permission to make mistakes and learn from them, for it is through these experiences that personal growth and resilience are cultivated.

Adapting to the demands of motherhood also involves nurturing your relationships, both with your child and with your partner. Take time to bond with your baby, engaging in activities that promote connection and attachment. Cherish the precious moments of bonding through breastfeeding, skin-to-skin contact, and gentle interactions. Nurture your relationship with your partner by maintaining open communication, expressing your needs and concerns, and finding opportunities for quality time together.

As you adapt to the demands of motherhood, remember to be patient and kind to yourself. Give yourself permission to make adjustments, seek support when needed, and celebrate your successes along the way. Embrace the transformative power of motherhood and the love that flows through this incredible journey. With each passing day, you will continue to grow, learn, and navigate the beautiful path of motherhood with grace and resilience.

Nurturing Yourself while Caring for Your Baby

Motherhood is a beautiful and rewarding journey that involves caring for your baby with love and dedication. Amidst the joy and fulfillment of nurturing your little one, it is equally important to prioritize self-care and nurture yourself. Taking care of your own well-being not only benefits you but also enhances your ability to care for your baby.

Here are some ways to nurture yourself while caring for your baby:

1. Prioritize Rest and Sleep:
Sleep deprivation is a common challenge for new mothers. While it may seem difficult to find time for rest, prioritize getting enough sleep whenever possible. Take short naps during the day when your baby is asleep, and consider asking for support from your partner, family, or friends to help with nighttime feedings. Remember, your body needs rest to recover and replenish energy.

2. Nourish Your Body:
Proper nutrition is essential for your well-being and overall energy levels. Aim to consume a balanced diet that includes nutritious foods such as fruits, vegetables, lean proteins, whole grains, and healthy fats. Stay hydrated by drinking plenty of water throughout the day. Consider meal prepping or accepting help from loved ones

to ensure you have nourishing meals readily available.

3. Find Moments for Self-Care:
Even in the midst of caring for your baby, find small moments for self-care. Take a relaxing bath, indulge in a favorite hobby, read a book, or listen to calming music. Use these moments to reconnect with yourself and recharge your emotional well-being. Self-care doesn't have to be time-consuming; even a few minutes of intentional self-care can make a difference.

4. Engage in Gentle Exercise:
Physical activity can help boost your mood, energy levels, and overall well-being. Engage in gentle exercises, such as walking, yoga, or postpartum exercises specifically designed for new mothers. Check with your healthcare provider before starting any exercise routine and listen to your body's cues to avoid overexertion.

5. Connect with Others:
Nurturing yourself involves maintaining social connections and seeking support from others. Connect with fellow mothers, join parenting groups, or attend local community events for parents. These connections provide opportunities to share experiences, seek advice, and form friendships with others who understand the joys and challenges of motherhood.

6. Practice Mindfulness and Relaxation:
Take moments throughout the day to practice mindfulness and relaxation techniques. Deep breathing exercises, meditation, or guided imagery can help reduce stress, promote a sense of calm, and improve overall well-being. Incorporate these practices into your daily routine, even if it's for a few minutes at a time.

7. Ask for Help:
Remember that it's okay to ask for help when you need it. Reach out to your partner,

family members, or friends for support. Whether it's help with household chores, childcare, or simply providing a listening ear, accepting help can alleviate some of the pressures and allow you time for self-care.

8. Embrace Imperfection:
Motherhood can be demanding, and it's important to let go of the expectation of being a perfect mother. Embrace the imperfections and learn to celebrate small victories. Give yourself grace and acknowledge that you are doing the best you can. Allow yourself to grow, learn, and adapt as you navigate the beautiful journey of motherhood.

Remember, nurturing yourself is not a luxury but a necessity. By prioritizing self-care and nurturing your own well-being, you will have more energy, patience, and love to share with your baby. Taking care of yourself is an essential part of being a loving and present mother. Embrace this precious time with your baby while also nurturing your own body, mind, and spirit.

Building Confidence in Your Parenting Abilities

Becoming a parent is a transformative experience that can bring immense joy, but it can also come with feelings of uncertainty and self-doubt. However, it is important to remember that you have the innate ability to be a wonderful parent to your child. Building confidence in your parenting abilities is a journey that involves self-reflection, learning, and embracing your unique strengths. Here are some strategies to help you build confidence in your parenting abilities:

1. Embrace Your Intuition:
Trust your instincts and embrace your intuition as a parent. You know your child best, and your instincts can guide you in making decisions that are in their best

interest. Pay attention to your gut feelings and give yourself permission to follow them. Over time, as you witness the positive outcomes of your intuitive choices, your confidence will grow.

2. Educate Yourself:
Knowledge is empowering. Take the time to educate yourself about various aspects of parenting, such as child development, nutrition, discipline techniques, and communication strategies. Read books, attend parenting classes, and seek reliable resources to expand your understanding. The more informed you are, the more confident you will feel in making informed decisions for your child.

3. Seek Support and Guidance:
Building confidence in your parenting abilities is not a solitary journey. Surround yourself with a supportive network of family, friends, and fellow parents who can offer guidance, share their experiences, and

provide reassurance. Join parent support groups, participate in online forums, or seek professional advice when needed. Remember, seeking support is a sign of strength, not weakness.

4. Reflect on Your Strengths:
Take time to reflect on your unique strengths as a parent. Identify the qualities and skills that you possess, such as patience, empathy, or creativity. Acknowledge the positive moments and successes you have had as a parent, no matter how small they may seem. Recognize that you are capable of providing love, care, and guidance to your child in your own special way.

5. Learn from Mistakes:
Parenting is a learning process, and making mistakes is a natural part of that journey. Instead of dwelling on perceived failures, view them as opportunities for growth and learning. Reflect on what went wrong, identify the lesson, and make adjustments

for the future. Remember that everyone makes mistakes, and it is through these experiences that we become more resilient and compassionate parents.

6. Practice Self-Compassion:
Parenting can be challenging, and it is important to be kind and gentle with yourself. Acknowledge that you are doing the best you can with the resources and knowledge you have. Embrace self-compassion and let go of the unrealistic expectations of being a perfect parent. Celebrate your successes, big or small, and give yourself permission to learn and grow along the way.

7. Celebrate Your Bond with Your Child:
Take the time to cherish and celebrate the unique bond you share with your child. Notice the moments of connection, love, and joy that you experience together. These precious moments affirm your deep connection and serve as a reminder that

you are an important and loving presence in your child's life.

8. Practice Mindfulness:
Mindfulness can help you cultivate confidence in your parenting abilities by allowing you to be fully present and engaged in the moment. Practice being mindful during interactions with your child, observing their cues, and responding with intention and love. By staying present and attuned to your child's needs, you will strengthen your bond and develop a deeper understanding of your own capabilities as a parent.

Remember that building confidence in your parenting abilities is a continuous process. It takes time, patience, and self-reflection. Trust yourself, embrace your unique journey as a parent, and know that you are capable of providing love, care, and guidance to your child.

Chapter 12: Celebrating Your Journey

Becoming a parent is a remarkable journey filled with ups and downs, challenges and triumphs, and an abundance of love and joy. As you navigate the beautiful path of parenthood, it is important to pause, reflect, and celebrate the milestones, growth, and incredible moments that shape your journey. Celebrating your journey as a parent is not only a way to acknowledge your achievements but also a means of cultivating gratitude, finding strength in difficult times, and cherishing the precious memories created along the way.

In this chapter, we will explore the importance of celebrating your journey as a parent and discover various ways to honor and embrace the experiences that make your journey unique. From the first moments of anticipation to the everyday joys and challenges, each step holds significance and deserves to be acknowledged and celebrated.

Parenthood is a transformative experience that stretches you in ways you never imagined. It is a journey of self-discovery, personal growth, and unconditional love. By taking the time to celebrate your journey, you not only honor yourself as a parent but also create a positive and nurturing environment for your child. Celebration is a powerful tool that can deepen your connection with your child, strengthen your bond as a family, and infuse your parenting journey with gratitude and positivity.

Reflecting on the Incredible Journey of Pregnancy

Reflecting on the incredible journey of pregnancy allows you to pause, acknowledge, and celebrate the transformative experience you have undergone. It is a time of self-discovery, growth, and awe-inspiring moments that shape you as an expectant mother. By taking the time to reflect on the different aspects of your journey, you can deepen your connection with your baby, cultivate gratitude, and gain a deeper appreciation for the miracle of life.

1. Embracing the Miracle of Life: Pregnancy is a profound and miraculous process that brings forth new life. Reflecting on this journey helps you acknowledge the awe-inspiring nature of pregnancy. From the moment of conception to the development of your baby's tiny limbs and organs, you can marvel at the intricate workings of the human body and the miracle of creation.

2. Appreciating the Physical Changes: Pregnancy brings about remarkable physical changes as your body adapts and

nurtures the growing life within you. Reflect on the changes you have experienced, such as the expansion of your belly, the sensation of your baby's movements, and the unique changes in your skin, hair, and nails. Embrace these changes as signs of the incredible journey you are on.

3. Honoring the Emotional Rollercoaster: Pregnancy is a time of heightened emotions. Reflecting on your emotional journey allows you to acknowledge the range of feelings you have experienced, from excitement and joy to anxiety and vulnerability. Recognize that these emotions are a natural part of the process and a testament to the love and connection you already have with your baby.

4. Celebrating Milestones: Pregnancy is marked by various milestones that deserve celebration. Reflect on the milestones you have reached, such as hearing your baby's heartbeat for the first time, feeling their first

kicks, or seeing their tiny form on an ultrasound. These milestones represent the progress and growth of your baby and offer moments of profound joy and anticipation.

5. Nurturing the Bond: Pregnancy provides a unique opportunity to bond with your baby before they even enter the world. Reflect on the moments of connection you have experienced, whether it's through gentle touches, talking or singing to your baby, or simply taking time to rest and be present with them. Embrace the power of this bond and allow it to deepen your connection with your growing baby.

6. Gratitude for the Journey: Take a moment to express gratitude for the journey of pregnancy. Reflect on the privilege of carrying life, the support you have received from loved ones and healthcare professionals, and the strength and resilience you have demonstrated along the way. Cultivating gratitude allows you to find

joy and appreciation in each step of the journey.

7. Documenting Memories: Consider documenting your pregnancy journey through photographs, journaling, or creating a scrapbook. Capture the special moments, milestones, and reflections that have shaped your experience. These memories will serve as a precious keepsake and a way to share your journey with your child in the future.

Reflecting on the incredible journey of pregnancy allows you to honor the beauty, challenges, and growth that have shaped your path to motherhood. It is a time of self-reflection, gratitude, and celebration. Embrace the unique experience of pregnancy and cherish the memories that will accompany you as you prepare to welcome your baby into the world.

Honoring the Challenges and Triumphs

Honoring the challenges and triumphs of pregnancy is an essential part of reflecting on your journey and celebrating the strength and resilience you have demonstrated. Pregnancy is not without its difficulties, both physical and emotional, but it is also a time of personal growth, empowerment, and triumphs. By acknowledging and honoring both the challenges and triumphs, you can gain a deeper appreciation for your journey and the incredible woman you have become.

1. Recognizing the Physical Challenges: Pregnancy can bring a range of physical challenges, such as morning sickness, fatigue, discomfort, and changes in your body. Reflect on the times when you felt physically challenged and remember the strength it took to endure and overcome them. Each day, you faced the physical demands of pregnancy with courage and determination.

2. Navigating Emotional Rollercoasters: Pregnancy is often accompanied by a rollercoaster of emotions. Hormonal changes, fears, anxieties, and mood swings can create emotional challenges. Take a moment to honor the times when you faced these emotional struggles head-on, sought support when needed, and found ways to manage and balance your emotions. Your ability to navigate these challenges demonstrates your emotional resilience.

3. Overcoming Pregnancy-Related Concerns: Pregnancy can bring about various concerns and worries, such as health complications, birth complications, or the well-being of your baby. Reflect on the times when you faced these concerns with courage and sought the necessary support and information to address them. Each step you took to address and overcome these challenges showcases your strength and determination as an expectant mother.

4.   Celebrating   Milestones   and Achievements: Pregnancy is filled with milestones and achievements that deserve celebration. From completing each trimester to reaching important prenatal appointments, each milestone represents progress and growth. Take time to honor these milestones and acknowledge the strength and perseverance it took to reach them. Celebrate the small victories as well, such as adopting healthy habits or managing discomforts.

5. Embracing Personal Growth: Pregnancy is a transformative time that fosters personal growth. Reflect on the ways in which you have grown as an individual throughout your pregnancy journey. This can include developing patience, nurturing a stronger sense of empathy, learning to trust your instincts, or embracing your own body and self-image. Celebrate the personal growth you have experienced and recognize the

positive impact it will have on your journey into motherhood.

6. Seeking Support and Building Resilience: Pregnancy often requires seeking support and building resilience. Reflect on the times when you reached out for guidance, leaned on your support system, or sought professional help when needed. Acknowledge the strength it took to ask for support and recognize the resilience you have developed as a result. Celebrate the connections and relationships that have uplifted you on this journey.

7. Cultivating Self-Care and Prioritizing Your Well-being: Pregnancy necessitates self-care and prioritizing your well-being. Reflect on the times when you made conscious efforts to take care of yourself, both physically and emotionally. Celebrate the moments when you listened to your body, rested when needed, nourished yourself with healthy choices, and engaged

in activities that brought you joy and relaxation. Recognize the importance of self-care in nurturing yourself and your growing baby.

Honoring the challenges and triumphs of pregnancy is an opportunity to celebrate your resilience, strength, and personal growth. It is a testament to the incredible journey you are undertaking and the powerful woman you are becoming as you prepare to bring new life into the world. Embrace the challenges, celebrate the triumphs, and carry the lessons learned throughout your journey into the next chapter of motherhood.

Embracing the Love and Joy that Motherhood Brings

Embracing the love and joy that motherhood brings is a beautiful and transformative aspect of the journey. As you prepare to welcome your baby into the world, it is important to reflect on the immense love and joy that awaits you. Motherhood is a profound experience that will fill your heart with unconditional love unlike any other.

1. Anticipating the Bond: Motherhood is a journey that deepens the bond between you and your baby. Reflect on the anticipation of holding your little one in your arms for the first time, the joy of feeling their tiny fingers wrap around yours, and the overwhelming love that will wash over you. Embrace the excitement and joy that comes with the anticipation of the precious bond you will share with your baby.

2. Cherishing Everyday Moments: Motherhood is filled with countless special moments that will bring you immense joy. Reflect on the simple yet profound moments of connection, like feeling your baby's gentle kicks, hearing their hiccups, or experiencing their first smiles. These everyday moments

are precious and will fill your heart with immeasurable joy and gratitude.

3. Creating Lasting Memories: Motherhood offers an opportunity to create cherished memories that will last a lifetime. Reflect on the memories you will make, from capturing your baby's first milestones to creating family traditions and experiencing new adventures together. Embrace the joy of being present in these moments and capturing them through photographs, journals, or other means to preserve the memories for years to come.

4. Finding Joy in the Little Things: Motherhood invites you to find joy in the simplest of things. Reflect on the joy that comes from snuggling your baby, singing lullabies, or watching them explore the world with curiosity. Embrace the wonder and delight that your little one will bring into your life and revel in the beauty of the ordinary

moments that become extraordinary through their eyes.

5. Nurturing and Growing Together: Motherhood is a journey of mutual growth and nurturing. Reflect on the joy of witnessing your baby's growth and development, celebrating their milestones, and supporting them as they explore the world. Embrace the opportunity to nurture and guide your child, knowing that your love and care will play a fundamental role in shaping their future.

6. Cultivating Gratitude: Motherhood is an invitation to cultivate gratitude for the precious gift of your child. Reflect on the gratitude you feel for the opportunity to experience the love, joy, and challenges that come with being a mother. Embrace a daily practice of gratitude, acknowledging the blessings and joys that motherhood brings, even amidst the inevitable ups and downs.

7. Embracing the Journey: Motherhood is a journey that unfolds with each passing day. Reflect on the beauty of this journey, knowing that it will have its highs and lows, its challenges and rewards. Embrace the unknown and trust in your ability to navigate the path ahead with love, resilience, and an open heart.

Embracing the love and joy that motherhood brings allows you to fully immerse yourself in the transformative experience of being a mother. It is a journey that will fill your heart with love, bring immeasurable joy, and shape you into the incredible mother you are meant to be. Cherish the moments, embrace the love, and allow the joy of motherhood to permeate every aspect of your life.

As you embark on the journey of celebrating your own experiences as a parent, remember that each step, no matter how challenging or mundane it may seem, contributes to the growth and strength you cultivate along the way. By taking the time to reflect, express gratitude, and connect with others, you honor the transformative power of parenthood and create a legacy of love and celebration for your child.

So, embrace this chapter as an invitation to celebrate your journey. May it inspire you to cherish the remarkable moments, find beauty in the ordinary, and create a tapestry of memories that reflect the depth of your love and dedication as a parent.

Conclusion

In conclusion, "The Confident Mama-To-Be: Navigating Pregnancy with Ease" is a comprehensive guidebook designed to support and empower expectant mothers on their pregnancy journey. Throughout the book, we have explored various topics that are essential for navigating pregnancy with confidence, ease, and joy.

From discovering the miracle of pregnancy to embracing the physical and emotional changes, building a support network, and nurturing your body, we have delved into the fundamental aspects of pregnancy. We have explored the importance of cultivating emotional well-being, creating a safe and nurturing environment, and bonding with your baby. We have also discussed the art of pregnancy fashion, navigating the medical maze, and preparing for labor, delivery, and postpartum.

Throughout the book, we have emphasized the significance of self-care, self-compassion, and the importance of building a strong support system. We have encouraged expectant mothers to trust their instincts, make informed decisions, and advocate for their birth preferences. We have highlighted the beauty of the journey, celebrated the challenges and triumphs, and explored the love and joy that motherhood brings.

As you embark on your own pregnancy journey, remember that you are not alone. This book serves as a guide and companion, providing you with knowledge, guidance, and inspiration. Trust yourself, listen to your body, and embrace the incredible journey that lies ahead.

May this book empower you to navigate pregnancy with confidence, grace, and ease. May it provide you with the tools and insights needed to overcome challenges, make informed choices, and cultivate a deep connection with your baby. Remember that you are a remarkable woman, capable of embracing the transformative experience of pregnancy and motherhood.

May you approach each day with gratitude, resilience, and a sense of wonder. May you find joy in the smallest of moments and cherish the milestones that mark this extraordinary journey. And above all, may you embrace the confident mama-to-be within you, knowing that you are equipped with the strength, wisdom, and love to navigate this beautiful journey with grace.

Congratulations, mama-to-be, on embarking on this incredible journey of pregnancy. Trust yourself, honor your unique path, and may your journey be filled with love, joy, and an abundance of beautiful memories.